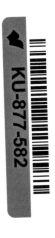
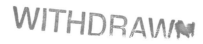

Serono Symposia International Foundation

Dictionary of Multiple Sclerosis

Dedication

To patients and their relatives who attended neurology clinics in the UK for years with the hope they might receive new innovative disease-modulating treatments readily available elsewhere in Europe, North America and Australia. Their fortitude, patience and courage when denied access to these effective treatments, often in the face of unpleasant relapses and accumulating disability, was remarkable and inspiring. They deserved better.

LDB

Serono Symposia International Foundation

Dictionary of Multiple Sclerosis

Editor-in-Chief
Lance D Blumhardt MD FRCP
Professor Emeritus of Clinical Neurology

Associate Editor
Xia Lin PhD
Research Fellow in Clinical Neurology

Division of Clinical Neurology
University Hospital
Queen's Medical Centre
University of Nottingham
Nottingham, United Kingdom

Section Editors

CS Constantinescu

G Giovannoni

JF Kurtzke

DKB Li

PS Sorensen

GC Ebers

J Kesselring

H Lassmann

C Liu

†JN Whitaker

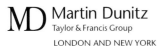

Martin Dunitz
Taylor & Francis Group
LONDON AND NEW YORK

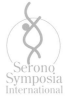

Serono
Symposia
International

© 2004 Martin Dunitz, an imprint of the Taylor & Francis Group plc

First published in the United Kingdom in 2004
by Martin Dunitz, an imprint of the Taylor & Francis Group plc, 11 New Fetter
Lane, London EC4P 4EE

Tel.: +44 (0) 20 7583 9855
Fax.: +44 (0) 20 7842 2298
E-mail: info@dunitz.co.uk
Website: http://www.dunitz.co.uk

Although every effort has been made to ensure that drug doses and other
information are presented accurately in this publication, the ultimate
responsibility rests with the prescribing physician. Neither the publishers, the
authors nor Serono Symposia International Foundation (Rome, Italy) shall be
held liable for errors or for any consequences arising out of the use of the
information contained herein.

A CIP record for this book is available from the British Library.

ISBN 1-85317-866-7

Distributed in the USA by
Fulfilment Center
Taylor & Francis
10650 Toebben Drive
Independence, KY 41051, USA
Toll Free Tel.: +1 800 634 7064
E-mail: taylorandfrancis@thomsonlearning.com

Distributed in Canada by
Taylor & Francis
74 Rolark Drive
Scarborough, Ontario M1R 4G2, Canada
Toll Free Tel.: +1 877 226 2237
E-mail: tal_fran@istar.ca

Distributed in the rest of the world by
Thomson Publishing Services
Cheriton House
North Way
Andover, Hampshire SP10 5BE, UK
Tel.: +44 (0)1264 332424
E-mail: salesorder.tandf@thomsonpublishingservices.co.uk

Composition by Wearset Ltd, Boldon, Tyne & Wear

Printed and bound in Great Britain by The Cromwell Press Ltd,
Trowbridge, Wilts.

Contents

Contributors

Lance D Blumhardt MD FRCP
Professor Emeritus of Clinical
Neurology
Division of Clinical Neurology
University Hospital
Queen's Medical Centre
University of Nottingham
Nottingham NG7 2UH
United Kingdom

Chris S Constantinescu MD PhD
Head (Acting) and Clinical Senior
Lecturer
Division of Clinical Neurology
University Hospital
Queen's Medical Centre
University of Nottingham
Nottingham NG7 2UH
United Kingdom

George C Ebers MD FRCPC
Action Research Professor of Clinical
Neurology
Head, Department of Clinical
Neurology
Medical Sciences Division
Oxford University
Oxford OX2 6HE
United Kingdom

Gavin Giovannoni MBBCh FCP PhD
Senior Clinical Lecturer in
Neuroimmunology
Institute of Neurology
University College London
Queen Square
London WC1N 3BG
United Kingdom

Jürg Kesselring MD
Professor of Neurology and
Neurorehabilitation
University of Bern and Zürich
Head of Neurology
Klinik Valens
Valens CH–7317
Switzerland

John F Kurtzke MD
Professor of Neurology
Georgetown University School of
Medicine
Chief, Neuroepidemiology Section
Veterans Affairs Medical Center
Washington, DC 20422
USA

Hans Lassmann MD
Head, Division of Neuroimmunology
Brain Research Institute
University of Vienna
A–1090 Vienna
Austria

David KB Li MD FRCPC
Professor of Radiology
University of British Columbia
UBC Hospital – Department of
Radiology
Vancouver
British Columbia V6T 2B5
Canada

Xia Lin PhD
Research Fellow in Clinical Neurology
Division of Clinical Neurology
University Hospital
Queen's Medical Centre
University of Nottingham
Nottingham NG7 2UH
United Kingdom

Clarence Liu MA MRCP DM
Consultant Neurologist
The Royal London and Homerton
University Hospitals
London E1 1BB
United Kingdom

Per S Sorensen MD DMSc
Professor of Neurology
MS Research Unit
Department of Neurology
Copenhagen University Hospital
Righospitalet
DK–2100 Copenhagen
Denmark

†**John N Whitaker** MD
Chairman
Department of Neurology
University of Alabama at Birmingham
Birmingham, AL 25294–7340
USA

Foreword

Approximately 2.5 million people worldwide have multiple sclerosis (MS), a chronic, incurable and often disabling illness of the central nervous system. There are many more people who are affected by MS indirectly each day, as they provide support, either professionally or personally, to those living with MS.

It is essential that reliable and factual information about MS is accessible to ensure that all the people affected by the disorder can keep up to date with the latest developments in the field. However, while an ever-increasing amount of information is made available from a wide variety of sources, it is often presented in a medical jargon that can be confusing or difficult to understand. Therefore the *Dictionary of Multiple Sclerosis* is a very welcome addition to the literature.

The *Dictionary* defines all the main terms relating to MS and provides a much-needed key to the more complex texts available. It is an invaluable reference tool for both clinicians and paraclinical personnel, as well as for those personally affected by MS.

Jürg Kesselring, Chair
International Medical and Scientific Board of MSIF

Christine Purdy, Chief Executive
Multiple Sclerosis International Federation (MSIF)

Preface

Over many years I have seen young research workers, trainee (and not so trainee) neurologists, doctors, nurses, pharmaceutical representatives and patients struggle to come to terms with the vast knowledge base and terminology of multiple sclerosis (MS). Any of these may encounter (and need to understand) terms from clinical neurology, genetics, molecular biology, biochemistry, immunology, pathology, radiology, clinical trial methodology, pathogenesis, therapeutics and epidemiology. The ever-expanding list of publications and terminologies means that few individuals can quickly master all aspects of MS.

We did not set out to write a textbook – there are many excellent examples available – but instead aimed at the concept of a desktop reference resource or 'dictionary' that could provide a handy entrée to a term supported by one or two key references. The difficulties inherent include the huge and expanding terminology – too bulky in fact for one dictionary - and the (usually arbitrary) decision on sensible 'cut-off points' for definitions. Nevertheless, we have had a stab at selecting a sample of terms that we hope might be useful to a greater or lesser extent for anyone interested in MS. In particular, we were aiming at young clinicians entering this field, for neurologists without (or perhaps even with) a special interest in MS, paraclinical personnel, and patients and relatives who are increasingly interested in all aspects of their disease.

I have been fortunate to have the help of Dr Xia Lin, whose initial drafting of terms and definitions kick-started the project, and of a panel of invited international experts who checked lists under specific headings and advised on inclusion or exclusion of terms and their definitions. I am indebted to their efforts, although ultimately the final responsibility for an apparently arbitrary choice of terms, for any off-target, over-simplified or inaccurate definitions, must lie with the editor. Any constructive criticism or contributions that may improve and enhance the next edition will of course be only too welcome!

I hope that this compilation of terms and tools for describing and measuring different aspects of MS might prove to be useful for someone, somewhere. If it helps to save just a few minutes, throw some light on just one strange term, suggest one reference that proves helpful, or facilitates access to a particular clinical rating scale, I will consider my time well spent.

LDB

Waiheke Island
October 2003

Acknowledgements

Special thanks are due to Gavin Giovannoni and Jia Newcombe at the Institute of Neurology, Queen Square, London, for providing valuable original illustrations, to Jean-Pierre Malkowski, Philippe Fonjallaz, Sophie Macchitella-Froissart of Serono International SA (Geneva) for their relentless commitment and assistance, and to Maria Grazia Calì, President, Serono Symposia International Foundation (Rome), for providing essential financial support. In addition, I wish to express my gratitude to Christine Purdy, Chief Executive, Multiple Sclerosis International Federation (MSIF) and to Jürg Kesselring (MSIF) for their close collaboration. Finally, I would like to acknowledge Martin Dunitz for backing the concept and Pete Stevenson (Taylor & Francis Medical) for his persistent devotion.

Figures and Tables – Sources and Acknowledgements

Figures 2, 4A, 16A and 20: Reproduced with permission from Alberts B, Bray D, Lewis J et al. , eds. *Molecular Biology of the Cell*, 3rd edition. London: Garland Publishing, 1994.

Figure 8: Reproduced with permission from Purves D, Augustine GJ, Fitzpatrick D et al., eds. *Neuroscience*. Sunderland, MA, USA: Sinauer Associates Inc. Publishers, 1997.

Figures 12.1 and 17: Reproduced from Matthews WB, Martyn CN, Allen IV et al. *McAlpine's Multiple Sclerosis* 2nd edition. Edinburgh: Churchill Livingstone, 1991, with permission from Elsevier.

Figures 12.2–5: Reproduced with permission from Lublin FD, Reingold SC, for the National Multiple Sclerosis Society (USA) Advisory Committee on Clinical Trials of New Agents in Multiple Sclerosis. Defining the clinical course of multiple sclerosis: results of an international survey. *Neurology* 1996; **46**: 907–10.

Figures 21 and 23: Reproduced with permission from Hohlfeld R. Biotechnological agents for the immunotherapy of multiple sclerosis. Principles, problems and perspectives. *Brain* 1997; **120**: 865–916.

Table 1: Adapted with permission from Brew B, Sidtis J, Petito CK, Price RW. The neurologic complications of AIDS and human immunodeficiency virus infection. In: Plum F, ed. *Advances in Contemporary Neurology*. Philadelphia, PA, USA: Davis, 1988.

Tables 2 and 5: Reproduced with permission from Hohlfeld R. Biotechnological agents for the immunotherapy of multiple sclerosis. Principles, problems and perspectives. *Brain* 1997; **120**: 865–916.

Table 3: Adapted with permission from McFarland HF, Martin R, McFarlin DE. Genetic influences in multiple sclerosis. In: Raine CS, McFarland HF, Tourtellotte WW, eds. *Multiple Sclerosis: Clinical and pathogenetic basis*. London: Chapman & Hall Medical, 1997: 205–19.

Tables 4 and 20: Adapted with permission from Paty D. Interferon beta-1b. In: Hawkins CP, Wolinsky JS, eds. *Principles of Treatments in Multiple Sclerosis*. Oxford: Butterworth Heinemann, 2000.

Table 7: Reproduced with permission from McDonald WI, Compston A, Edan G et al. Recommended diagnostic criteria for multiple sclerosis: guidelines from the International Panel on the Diagnosis of Multiple Sclerosis. *Ann Neurol* 2001; **50**: 121–7.

Table 8: Reproduced with permission from McDonald WI, Halliday AM. Diagnosis and classification of multiple sclerosis. *Br Med Bull* 1977; **33**: 4–9.

Table 9: Reproduced with permission from Poser CM, Paty DW, Scheinberg L et al. New diagnostic criteria for multiple sclerosis: guidelines for research protocols. *Ann Neurol* 1983; **13**: 227–31.

Table 10: Reproduced with permission from Schumacher GA, Beebe G, Kebler RF et al. Problems of experimental trials of therapy in multiple sclerosis: report by the panel on the evaluation of experimental trials of therapy in multiple sclerosis. *Ann NY Acad Sci* 1965; **122**: 552–68.

Table 12: Adapted with permission from Polman CK. *Multiple Sclerosis: The guide to treatment and management*. New York, NY, USA: Demos, 2001.

Table 17: Adapted with permission from Comi G et al. Measuring evoked responses in multiple sclerosis. *Mult Scler* 1999; **5**: 263–7.

Table 18: Reproduced with permission from Poser CM, ed. *An Atlas of Multiple Sclerosis*. London: Parthenon Publishing, 1998.

Table 19: Reproduced with permission from Blumhardt LD. Interferon beta-1a. In: Hawkins CP, Wolinsky JS, eds. *Principles of Treatments in Multiple Sclerosis*. Oxford: Butterworth Heinemann, 2000.

Table 21: Adapted from Edan G, Morrisey S. Mitoxantrone. In: Hawkins CP, Wolinsky JS, eds. *Principles of Treatments in Multiple Sclerosis*. Oxford: Butterworth Heinemann, 2000.

Table 23: Adapted with permission from Poser CM. The epidemiology of multiple sclerosis: a general overview. *Ann Neurol* 1994; **36**(suppl 2): S180–93.

Abbreviations

ACE	angiotensin converting enzyme
ACTH	adrenocorticotropic hormone
ADC	apparent diffusion coefficient
ADEM	acute disseminated encephalomyelitis
AI	Ambulation Index
AIDS	acquired immunodeficiency syndrome
AION	anterior ischaemic optic neuropathy
Alb	albumin
APC	antigen-presenting cell
APL	altered peptide ligand
APS	antiphospholipid syndrome
AUC	area under the curve
BAEP	brainstem auditory evoked potential
BBB	blood–brain barrier
BCG	bacille Calmette–Guerin
BOD	burden of disease
BTX	botulinum toxin
C	complement
CAM	cell adhesion molecule
CAMS	Cambridge Basic Multiple Sclerosis Score
CC	corpus callosum
CCT	central conduction time
CD	clinically definite
CD	cluster of differentiation (antigens)
2-CdA	2-chlorodeoxyadenosine
CHAMPS	Controlled High-Risk Subjects Avonex Multiple Sclerosis Prevention Study
CMCT	central motor conduction time
CNS	central nervous system
CP	clinically probable

CSF	cerebrospinal fluid
CSM	cervical spondylotic myelopathy
CTLA-4	cytotoxic T-lymphocyte-associated protein 4
CU	combined unique
Cys	cysteine
DNA	deoxyribonucleic acid
DSS	Disability Status Scale
DTPA	diethylenetriamine pentaacetic acid
EAE	experimental allergic encephalomyelitis
EDMUS-GS	European Database for Multiple Sclerosis Grading Scale
EDSS	Expanded Disability Status Scale
ELAM-1	endothelial leukocyte adhesion molecule-1
EP	evoked potential
ERP	event-related potential
ESR	erythrocyte sedimentation rate
ESS	Environmental Status Scale
ETOMS	Early Treatment of Multiple Sclerosis
EVIDENCE	Evidence for Interferon Dose Effect: European-North American Comparative Efficacy
FAMS	Functional Assessment of Multiple Sclerosis
FDA	Food and Drug Administration
FIM	Functional Independence Measure
FLAIR	fluid-attenuated inversion recovery
FSE	fast spin echo
GA	glatiramer acetate
GABA	γ-aminobutyric acid
Gd	gadolinium
Glu	glutamine
GNDS	Guy's Neurological Disability Scale
HIV	human immunodeficiency virus
HLA	human leukocyte antigen
9-HPT	Nine-Hole Peg Test
HRQL	Health-Related Quality of Life
5HT	5-hydroxytryptamine

HTLV-1	human T-lymphotropic virus type 1
Hz	Hertz
ICAM-1	intercellular cell adhesion molecule-1
IFN	interferon
Ig	immunoglobulin
IgG	immunoglobulin G
IgM	immunoglobulin M
IL	interleukin
INO	internuclear ophthalmoplegia
ISS	Incapacity Status Scale
IU	international unit
IVIg	intravenous immunoglobulin
kDa	kilodalton
KFS	Kurtzke Functional System Scores
LD	linkage disequilibrium
Leu	leucine
LFA	lymphocyte-function associated antigen
LP	lumbar puncture
LSD	laboratory-supported definite
LSP	laboratory-supported probable
LT	leukotriene
LT	lymphotoxin
LTM	long-term memory
mAB	monoclonal antibody
MAG	myelin-associated glycoprotein
MBP	myelin basic protein
MBPLM	myelin basic protein-like material
MEP	magnetic evoked motor potential
MEP	motor evoked potential
mg	milligram
mgm	milligram
MHC	major histocompatibility complex
MHz/T	megahertz/tesla
MIU	million international unit
MLF	medial longitudinal fasciculus

mm	millimetre
MNC	mononuclear cell
MOG	myelin oligodendrocyte glycoprotein
MOS	Medical Outcomes Study
MP-RAGE	magnetization prepared rapid acquisition gradient echo
MR	magnetic resonance
MRD	Minimal Record of Disability
MRI	magnetic resonance imaging
mRNA	messenger RNA
MRS	magnetic resonance spectroscopy
MS	multiple sclerosis
MSCRG	Multiple Sclerosis Collaborative Research Group
MSFC	Multiple Sclerosis Functional Composite
MSQLI	Multiple Sclerosis Quality of Life Inventory
MSQOL	Multiple Sclerosis Quality of Life
mtDNA	mitochondrial DNA
MT	magnetization transfer
MTI	magnetization transfer imaging
µg	microgram
NAA	N-acetyl aspartate
NABs	neutralizing antibodies
NAWM	normal appearing white matter
9-HPT	Nine-Hole Peg Test
NK	natural killer
NMR	nuclear magnetic resonance
NNT	number needed to treat
NO	nitric oxide
OAPR	onset-adjusted prevalence rate
OB	oligoclonal band
OCB	oligoclonal band
OG	oligodendrocyte
ON	optic neuritis
OPC	oligodendrocyte progenitor cell
OWIMS	Once Weekly Interferon for Multiple Sclerosis
P	probability
PASAT	paced auditory serial addition test

PD	proton density
PE	plasma exchange
PFA	polyunsaturated fatty acid
PLP	myelin proteolipid protein
PMLE	progressive multifocal leukencephalopathy
PMSA	primary multiple sclerosis affection
PP	primary progressive
PR	progressive—relapsing
PRISMS	Prevention of Relapses and Disability by Interferon beta-1a Subcutaneously in Multiple Sclerosis
QNE	Quantitative Neurological Examination
QoL	quality of life
RAPD	relative afferent pupillary defect
RBN	retrobulbar neuritis
RNA	ribonucleic acid
RP	relapsing—progressive
RR	relapsing—remitting
SD	standard deviation
SEP	somatosensory evoked potential
Ser	serine
SF-36	Short Form Health Survey
SLE	systemic lupus erythematosus
SMON	subacute myelo-optic neuritis
SNP	single nucleotide polymorphism
SNRS	Scripps Neurologic Rating Scale
SP	secondary progressive
SPECTRIMS	Secondary Progressive Efficacy Clinical Trial of Recombinant Interferon-beta-1a in Multiple Sclerosis
STIR	short inversion-time inversion-recovery sequence
T25W	timed 25-foot walk
Tc	T-cytotoxic cell
Tc1	T-cytotoxic 1 cell
Tc2	T-cytotoxic 2 cell
TCR	T-cell receptor
TE	echo time

TGF-β	transforming growth factor beta
TGSE	turbo gradient spin echo
Th	T-helper cell
Th0	T-helper 0 cell
Th1	T-helper 1 cell
Th2	T-helper 2 cell
Th3	T-helper 3 cell
THC	tetrahydrocannabinol
3D	three-dimensional
TLL	total lesion load
TNF	tumour necrosis factor
TNFR	tumour necrosis factor receptor
TPMT	thiopurine *S*-methyltransferase
TR	repetition time
TSE	turbo spin echo
UBO	unidentified bright object
UK	United Kingdom
UKNDS	United Kingdom Neurological Disability Scale
USA	United States of America
VCAM-1	vascular cell adhesion molecule-1
VEP	visual evoked potential
VLA	very late antigen
WHO	World Health Organization
WM	working memory

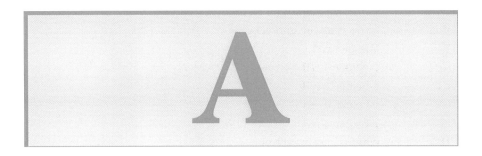

Achromatopsia   see *Dyschromatopsia.*

Acquired immunodeficiency syndrome (AIDS)   neurological syndrome caused by human immunodeficiency virus (HIV), which is characterized by an acquired and profound depression of cell-mediated immunity. Neurological manifestations range from subcortical dementia, through encephalitis, to full-blown AIDS syndrome comprising some or all of the complications listed in *Table 1.* Although white matter lesions on MRI closely resemble those of MS,[1] oligoclonal bands are rarely present in the CSF in AIDS. AIDS-related vascular myelopathy presents as progressive spastic paraparesis and sensory ataxia, but more closely resembles subacute combined degeneration of the spinal cord than MS.[2]

Active lesion   active MS lesions—as defined on MRI—are new, enlarging or recurrent lesions on T_2-weighted scans, or enhancing on T_1-weighted images.[3] Activity is due to recent, new or recurrent episodes of increased permeability of the blood–brain barrier with associated active inflammation and myelin breakdown.[4] [See also *T_2 active lesion* and *Gadolinium-enhancing lesion.*]

Activity limitation (WHO definition)   difficulty in the performance, accomplishment or completion of an activity at the level of the individual.[5] The difficulty encompasses all of the ways in which the doing of the activity may be affected. An activity limitation may range from a slight to severe deviation in terms of quality or quantity, in doing the activity in a manner or to the extent that is expected.

Acute disseminated encephalomyelitis (ADEM)   demyelinating disorder seen predominantly, but not exclusively, in children, and frequently preceded or accompanied by a clearly identifiable viral infection or inoculation.

1

Table 1 Neurological complications in HIV-1 infected patients

Brain
  Predominantly nonfocal
    AIDS dementia complex (subacute/chronic HIV encephalitis)
    Acute HIV-related encephalitis
    Cytomegalovirus encephalitis
    Varicella-zoster virus encephalitis
    Herpes simplex virus encephalitis
    Metabolic encephalopathies
  Predominantly focal
    Cerebral toxoplasmosis
    Primary CNS lymphoma
    Progressive multifocal leukoencephalopathy
    Cryptococcoma
    Brain abscess/tuberculoma
    Neurosyphilis (meningovascular)
    Vascular disorders – notably nonbacterial endocarditis and cerebral
      haemorrhages
    Associated with thrombocytopenia
Spinal cord
  Vacuolar myelopathy
  Herpes simplex or zoster myelitis
Meninges
  Aseptic meningitis (HIV)
  Cryptococcal meningitis
  Tuberculous meningitis
  Syphilitic meningitis
  Metastatic lymphomatous meningitis
Peripheral nerve and root
  Infectious
  Herpes zoster
  Cytomegalovirus lumbar polyradiculopathy
Virus- or immune-related
  Acute and chronic inflammatory HIV polyneuritis
  Mononeuritis multiplex
  Sensorimotor demyelinating polyneuropathy
  Distal painful sensory polyneuritis
Muscle
  Polymyositis and other myopathies (including drug-induced)

Adapted with permission.[8]

Characteristic stupor and coma at onset occur rarely in MS. ADEM typically is monophasic with widespread neurological abnormalities, including multifocal signs in the brain, spinal cord and optic nerves. Oligoclonal bands are usually absent or occur only transiently during the acute illness (once present, oligoclonal bands in MS usually persist). Cranial MRI may show rather symmetric and extensive lesions in the cerebral and cerebellar white matter and sometimes in the basal ganglia.[6] New lesions within 6 months' follow-up favour a diagnosis of MS rather than ADEM.[6,7]

Acute haemorrhagic leucoencephalomyelitis   more severe variant of acute disseminated encephalomyelitis (ADEM) in which the inflammatory reaction is associated with perivascular haemorrhages and severe brain oedema.[9] [See also *Acute disseminated encephalomyelitis*.]

Acute plaque (of MS)   ill-defined areas of pink, white or yellowish white matter in the CNS, many of which are visible macroscopically, in which the perivascular spaces, or the entire area, may be infiltrated by macrophages and lymphocytes, with endothelial cell activation, oedema, hypertrophic astrocytes, reduced oligodendrocytes and myelin, and variable degrees of remyelination often present in the centre of the lesion.[10] Four patterns of acute lesions have been described which share the T-cell- and macrophage-dominated inflammatory reaction: T-cell-mediated autoimmune encephalomyelitis (patterns I and II) and oligodendrocyte dystrophy (patterns III and IV).[11] [See *Figure 1*.]

Acute (subacute) myelopathy   partial or incomplete spinal cord lesions (e.g. a Brown–Séquard syndrome) are a common first presentation of demyelinating disease and carry a risk of developing 'clinical MS' from 42% to 80% during a mean follow-up period of 14–38 months.[12–15] The risk of conversion to CD MS is increased by the presence of HLA DR2, oligoclonal bands in the cerebrospinal fluid and the presence of disseminated brain lesions on MRI.[12–14]

Acute transverse myelopathy   see *Transverse myelitis*.

Acyclovir (Zovirax)   antiviral agent normally used to treat *herpes simplex* infections that may reduce the relapse rate in RR MS,[16] although larger trials are required for confirmation. A preliminary report of another small MRI study using valacyclovir, a prodrug of acyclovir, was negative.[17]

3

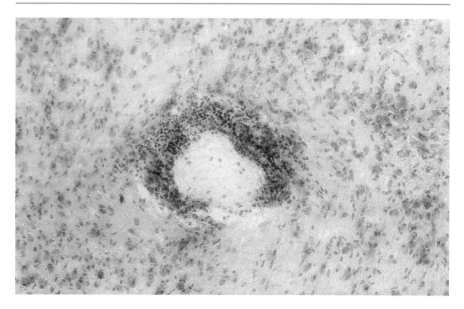

Figure 1 **Acute plaque** Red-stained macrophages containing lipids resulting from myelin breakdown surrounding a blood vessel with an inflammatory cuff of lymphocytes and macrophages. Oil red O and haematoxylin staining, magnification ×110. For full-colour version, please see accompanying CD. *(Courtesy of Dr J Newcombe, Institute of Neurology, London.)*

Adhesion molecules (cell adhesion molecules, CAMs) molecules mediating binding of cells with one another, or binding of cells with extracellular matrix components. CAMs include cell surface proteins that participate in leukocyte circulation, homing to tissues and inflammatory sites, and transendothelial migration. CAMs in endothelial cells participate and facilitate migration of lymphocytes across the blood–brain barrier in inflammatory autoimmune demyelination.[18] Adhesion molecules can be classified into several groups, including cadherins, selectins, integrins and Ig superfamily members [see *Table 2*]. Three adhesion proteins identified on human endothelial cells are vascular cell adhesion molecule-1 (VCAM-1), intracellular adhesion molecule-1 (ICAM-1) and endothelial leukocyte adhesion molecule (ELAM-1; E-selectin). Numerous studies report increased serum and cerebrospinal fluid levels of soluble VCAM-1, ICAM-1 and E-selectin in patients with MS.[19,20] [See *Figure 2*.]

Adrenocorticotropic hormone (ACTH) hormone produced by the pituitary gland that regulates the production of glucocorticosteroids by the adrenal

Table 2 Cell adhesion molecules

Name	Ligand	Expression (constitutive or induced)
Adhesion receptors of the selectin family		
L-selectin	Glycosylated mucinlike molecules	T, M, PMN
E-selectin	Sialylated mucinlike molecules	Activated EC
P-selectin	P-selectin glycoprotein ligand 1	P, activated EC
Mucin-like vascular addressins		
CD34	L-selectin	EC
GlyCAM-4	L-selectin	High endothelial venules
MadCAM-1	L-selectin, VLA-4	Mucosal lymphoid tissue venules
Adhesion receptors of the integrin family		
α4β1 (VLA-4)	VCAM, FN (CS-1), PP-HEV	T, B
α5β1 (VLA-5)	FN (RGD)	T, EC, epithelium, P
α6β1 (VLA-6)	LM	T, P
αLβ2 (LFA-1, CD11a/CD18)	ICAM-1, ICAM-2	Leukocytes
αMβ2 (MAC-1, CR3, CD11b/CD18)	ICAM-1, iC3b, FN, FX	M, PMN
αxβ2 (CR4, p150.95, CD11c/CD18)	FN, iC3b	M
α4β7	MAdCAM-1, VCAM	B, T
Adhesion receptors of the Ig superfamily		
ICAM-1 (CD54)	αLβ2, aMβ2	Activated EC, lymphocytes
ICAM-2 (CD102)	αLβ2	Resting EC
ICAM-3 (CD50)	αLβ2	APC
VCAM (CD106)	α4β1	Activated EC
LFA-2 (CD2)	LFA-3	T
LFA-3 (CD58)	CD2 (LFA-2)	Lymphocytes, APC

APC = antigen-presenting cell; CAM = cell adhesion molecule; CR = complement receptor; EC = endothelial cell; FN = fibronectin; HEV = high endothelial venule; ICAM = intercellular adhesion molecule; LFA = lymphocyte-function associated antigen; LM = laminin; M = monocyte/macrophage; P = platelet; PMN = polymorphonuclear leucocyte; PP = Peyer's plaque; VCAM = vascular cell adhesion molecule; VLA = very late antigen. Reproduced with permission.[21]

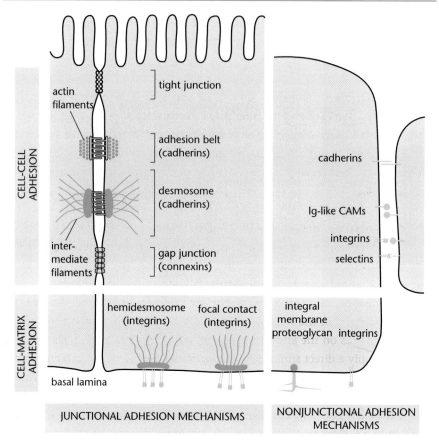

Figure 2 **Adhesion molecules (CAMs)** A summary of the junctional and nonjunctional adhesive mechanisms used by animal cells in binding to one another and to the extracellular matrix. Reproduced with permission.[21A]

gland. ACTH by injection was frequently used to treat acute exacerbations of MS in the past, but has been superseded by methylprednisolone and is no longer widely available. Nevertheless, there has been a continuing debate about the possible superiority of ACTH to glucocorticosteroids in increasing the rate of recovery from acute exacerbations.[22]

Adrenomyeloneuropathy adult variant of the X-linked disorder adrenoleucodystrophy with a slowly progressive neurological course characterized by spastic paraparesis, sometimes with cerebellar ataxia and intellectual deterioration in young adult males. Clinical clues include evidence of a peripheral neuropathy, increased skin pigmentation and thin hair. A definite diagnosis is established by demonstration of abnormal adrenal function and elevated serum levels of very long chain fatty acids. MRI abnormalities, when present, are very characteristic with symmetrical white matter lesions often in the posterior cerebral hemispheres.[23]

Affective disorders abnormal emotional states such as depression, anxiety or euphoria that are accompanied by disturbances of sleep and appetite, as well as by characteristic patterns of thought and behaviour. Patients with these disorders may complain of memory loss, poor concentration and changes to their usual ways of thinking [see also *Cognitive dysfunction* and *Depression*].

Afferent pupillary defect (RAPD, Marcus–Gunn pupil) detectable inter-ocular difference in the pupillary responses seen after unilateral optic nerve or retinal lesions. Any difference can be exaggerated by regular, rapid alternation of a light stimulus between the two eyes ('swinging torch test'). For example, after inducing a normal reflex constriction in the left eye (by shining a torch in the right eye), the torch is then swung across to apply a direct stimulus on the already contracted left pupil. The torch is then swung back to apply a direct stimulus to the right eye, and so on. An afferent pupillary defect is shown as a difference between the interacting direct and indirect pupillary responses on each side. The defect on the affected side may vary from a slight sluggishness of the direct vs indirect response to a reversed response, i.e. dilatation rather than constriction of the pupil on direct stimulation. The relative (i.e. interocular) amplitude of the 'escape' dilatation is a measure of the defective conduction in the abnormal eye. In one study, RAPD was positive in 32 (44%) out of 72 eyes with acute ON.[24]

Age-specific rate number of affected individuals related to a denominator confined to that proportion of the at-risk population with the same age. Age-specific rates may be calculated for incidence, prevalence or mortality. Similar calculations allow for comparisons between communities with different sex distributions [see also *Gender-specific rate(s)*].

Akinesia, paroxysmal sudden loss of power in the lower limbs described by patients as 'knees locking', 'legs collapsing', 'legs don't go', 'unexpected falls', often recurring several times a day and followed by rapid recovery.[660] May be difficult to diagnose when it is the presenting symptom.[661] The underlying mechanism is thought to be due to excessive discharges within an inhibitory path that serves the regulation of muscular tone.[660]

Albumin index   see *CSF/serum albumin quotient.*

Allele association   see *Linkage disequilibrium.*

Altered peptide ligands (APLs)   APLs are analogues of peptide determinants with one (or a few) substitutions at the amino acid positions essential for contact with T-cell receptors (TCR). The aim of using APLs in autoimmune disease is to induce anergy or tolerance to the inciting autoantigen. Two exploratory studies in MS using an APL of myelin basic protein were stopped prematurely, one because of an increase in disease activity[25] and the other because of hypersensitivity reactions.[26]

Amantadine hydrochloride   antiviral drug that is the first-line therapy for the treatment of MS-associated fatigue. It significantly improves fatigue in double-blind, placebo-controlled studies[27] and was superior to pemoline and placebo using a validated self-reported MS fatigue measure in a placebo-controlled randomized study.[28]

Ambulation Index (AI)   semi-quantitative tool that rates ambulation-related disability on an ordinal scale.[29] It specifies 10 grades ranging between 0 (normal) and 9 (wheelchair-bound and unable to transfer independently). The scale provides a more precise measure of ambulation than the EDSS in the range of scores between 4.0 and 6.0.[30] It is reported to have moderate to substantial inter-rater reliability,[31,32] but low responsiveness.[32] [See *Appendix* 3.]

Aminopyridine   potassium-channel blocking drug that has been reported to be effective in improving leg strength,[33] reducing fatigue[34,35] and increasing motor function in MS.[36] Significant side-effects include seizures.

Amitriptyline (Tryptizol)   tricyclic antidepressant with many useful symptomatic effects in MS. Helps to control emotional incontinence (pathological, exaggerated or inappropriate laughter or weeping), insomnia, nocturnal bladder control, dysaesthesiae and central pain. Often used in combination with anti-epileptic medication for pain and paraesthesiae.

Antegren   see *Anti-α 4 integrin antibody.*

Anterior ischaemic optic neuropathy (AION)   ischaemic infarction of the optic nerve head, characterized by abrupt visual loss. In some cases there

DICTIONARY OF MULTIPLE SCLEROSIS

may be progression over several days. Most subjects are over 50 years of age with associated vascular risk factors such as smoking, hypertension or diabetes. Younger patients with vasculitis may present with similar symptoms. Swelling of the optic disc and small, flamed-shaped haemorrhages on the optic disc are typical of AION.

Anti-α4 integrin antibody (Natalizumab, Antegren)   humanized monoclonal antibody (mAb) derived from a murine mAb raised against the human α4 integrin [see also *Integrin*]. It has inhibitory activity against α4 integrin-mediated cell adhesion both in vitro and in vivo[37] and suppresses EAE.[38] In a 24-week, phase II trial of RR and SP MS, the numbers of new active lesions on MRI were significantly reduced.[39] In a subsequent, 6-month phase II study there were marked reductions in the mean number of new lesions in Natalizumab groups: 9.6 per patient in the placebo group vs. 0.7 in the group given 3 mg Natalizumab/kg ($P < 0.001$) and 1.1 in the group given 6 mg Natalizumab/kg ($P < 0.001$). Twenty-seven patients in the placebo group had relapses, as compared with 13 in the 3 mg/kg Natalizumab group ($P = 0.02$) and 14 in the 6 mg/kg Natalizumab group ($P = 0.02$).[40] Further phase III studies of the effect of Antegren on MRI and clinical disease activity are currently under way.

Antibody   serum protein produced by terminally differentiated and activated B cells (plasma cells) that bind to epitopes on a given antigen [see also *B lymphocytes, Humoral immune response* and *Immunoglobulins*].

Anti-CD3 (OKT3)   IgG2a monoclonal antibody that stimulates release of lymphokines.[41] Unlikely to be used in the treatment of MS because of its toxicity.[42]

Anti-CD4   CD4+ helper T-lymphocytes may play an important role in the pathogenesis of MS. EAE in rodents or primates can be prevented by treatment with antibodies against CD4.[43] Intravenous treatment with anti-CD4 antibody in 71 patients resulted in a substantial reduction of both circulating CD4+ cells and clinical relapses, but this depletion was not associated with a significant decrease in disease activity or brain atrophy on MRI.[44,45] A possible explanation for the lack of efficacy of the anti-CD4 antibody may relate to its ability to cross the blood–brain barrier and the degree of depletion of CD4-positive cells.[45] A more marked depletion of CD4-positive cells in the circulation might be necessary to achieve positive results.

9

Anti-CD6 murine IgG monoclonal antibody against the T12 antigen present on most post-thymic T-lymphocytes. Disease activity appeared to stabilize in 6 of 12 patients with SP MS who received anti-CD6 therapy for 6 months.[46]

Anti-CD11/CD18 antibodies humanized mAb derived from a murine mAb raised against human CD11/CD18. Animals treated with anti-CD11/CD18 mAb showed a marked reduction in brain lesion area on MRI and improved neurological outcome.[47] A phase I trial of the humanized anti-CD11/CD18 antibodies in MS showed that the drug was well tolerated and both neurological and brain MRI parameters remained stable.[48]

Anti-CD52 see *Campath 1H.*

Antigen material (normally foreign) that is specifically bound by lymphocytes or antibodies. An antigen capable of eliciting an immune response is an immunogen.

Antigenic determinant site (epitope) on an antigen that elicits an immune response.

Antigen-presenting cells (APCs) host cells that display peptide–MHC complexes for recognition by T cells.[49] There are professional APCs (dendritic cells, macrophages) and facultative APCs that present antigen only in certain circumstances (for example, when they 'ectopically' or 'aberrantly' express MHC class II leading to autoimmune disease) [see also *Major histocompatibility complex* and *Trimolecular complex*].

Anti-inflammatory cytokines see *Cytokines.*

Antiphospholipid syndrome (APS) recently described entity characterized by deep venous thrombosis, multiple spontaneous miscarriages or strokes in young subjects in association with antiphospholipid antibodies.[50] A relapsing clinical syndrome has been described with a tendency for visual disturbances and multifocal white matter involvement, which may resemble the lesions of MS on MRI.[51] Anticardiolipin antibodies, coagulopathy, fever, raised ESR and weight loss may occur.

Antitumour necrosis factor (anti-TNF, cA2) treatment with anti-TNF improves animal models of MS, but in patients with MS, increases in MRI activity and worsening of CSF parameters have been observed.[52] [See also *Tumour necrosis factor alpha*.]

Apoptosis (programmed cell death) controlled autodigestion of a cell characterized by cytoskeletal disruption, cell shrinkage, membrane blebbing with nuclear condensation and fragmentation and, eventually, the formation of apoptotic bodies and the loss of mitochondrial function.[53]

Apparent diffusion coefficient (ADC) see *Diffusion-weighted imaging*.

Appropriateness term used to define whether the range of the construct measured within a study sample is similar to the range covered by the measurement instrument.[54] This reflects how relevant the instrument is to the population being examined. Appropriateness is usually assessed by examining distribution (i.e. ranges, means, SDs and floor and ceiling effects) for the measurement instrument.

Arcuate scotoma narrow slit-like curved defect of the visual field that results from damage to nerve-fibre bundles as they enter the papilla. The prevalence of arcuate scotomata in patients with MS has varied from 3.6%[55] to 76%[56] in different studies.

Area under the curve (AUC) statistical method of summarizing a time series that can be applied to any outcome measure. When applied to serial EDSS data over 2- or 3-year periods in RR MS, it has been considered statistically more powerful and clinically more meaningful than conventional methods of assessing disability changes.[57,58] It takes into account both transient and permanent disability worsening and thus summarizes the total disability (morbidity) experienced by patients during a study period.

Arnold–Chiari malformation congenital abnormality at the base of the brain characterized by variable protrusion of cerebellar tissue (cerebellar ectopia) into the upper cervical canal, displacement or angulation of the brain stem and underdevelopment of the posterior fossa.[59] Patients presenting in early or middle adult life with gait ataxia, spasticity of the limbs and nystagmus may be mistaken for MS, but distinguishing features include the presence of skeletal deformities of the neck, spine or skull in many patients, vertical nystagmus (unusual in MS) and characteristic abnormalities on MR images.

11

Ashworth Scale ordinal scale based on assessment of muscle tone. The most widely used clinical tool to quantify spasticity in MS.[60] It has an acceptable degree of inter-rater reliability.[61]

Asian MS characterized by a high incidence of optic–spinal involvement (e.g. 20–50% of MS patients in Japan).[62,63] Patients with Asian MS are thought to have fewer brain lesions on MRI and perhaps more gadolinium-enhancing spinal cord lesions than patients with Western-type MS.[64] Susceptibility to MS in Caucasians has repeatedly been shown to be associated with HLA-DRB1*1501-DQA1*0102-DQB1*0602,[65–67] whereas MS in Japan has shown an association with HLA-DPB1*0501.[68,69] Higher age of onset, higher EDSS scores and higher CSF cell and protein levels have also been reported in Asian patients.[68]

Association analysis technique designed to identify genetic markers with allele frequencies that differ in affected and unaffected individuals. A strong association of MS with HLA class II, particularly DR2 (DR15 /DRB1*1501) and with DQw6 has been reported. *Table 3* outlines the association between various HLA markers and MS. [See also *Human leukocyte antigen.*] The primary association in MS is in the class II region, but it is not yet clear with which gene. There are data favouring the DQ locus or an extended haplotype in this region which could include both DR and DQ. In animal models of autoimmune disease, homologues of both DR and DQ play roles.

Astrocyte star-shaped glial cell of the nervous system with diverse functions, including the provision of an architectural framework for neurons, a source of growth factor, a physiological role in conduction of the nerve impulse and participation in the response to injury.[80] Damage leads to synthesis of glial fibrils and scarring. [See *Figure 3.*]

Ataxia involvement of the cerebellum and cerebellar connections in the brain stem may lead to incoordination of one or more limbs, often associated with dysarthria and nystagmus. Midline cerebellar lesions may cause a truncal ataxia (failure of 'tandem walking' or heel–toe gait). Ataxia may also be caused by deafferentation and loss of joint position sense (proprioception) in a limb (sensory ataxia). Ataxia may also be a paroxysmal symptom [see also *Paroxysmal syndromes*].

Atrophy shrinkage or reduction in brain and spinal cord volume that results from loss of tissue. The pathological basis of atrophy in MS is unclear, but is

Table 3 Associations between HLA markers and MS

Population	Association	Reference
Mixed	DR2	66
Scandinavian	DR2	70
Arabian	DR4	71
Mexican	DRw6	72
Japanese	DRw6	73
Sardinian	DR4	74
Norwegian	Association particularly with DQB1 sequences	75
Norwegian	DQA1 with Glu at position 34	67

Swedish	Both RR and first-degree progressive—
	   DRw15, DQw6
	RR association with DRw17, DQw2
	First-degree progressive with DR4, DQw8
	   not confirmed
		76

Norwegian	Both RR and first-degree progressive—
	   DRw15, DQw6
	RR associated with DRw17, DQw2
	First-degree progressive with DR4, DQw8
	   not confirmed
	Association with DQB1 sequences or DQA1
	   Glu34 not confirmed
		77

French	Association with DR2 haplotype	

Canadians and
  mixed ethnic
  Caucasians
	(DRB1*1051, DQA1*0102, DQB1*0602)
	DQB1 sequences and DQA1 Glu34 linked to
	  haplotype not disease
	Association with DQB 1 Leu26 in French
	  Canadians but not mixed Caucasians
		78

Adapted and modified with permission.[79]

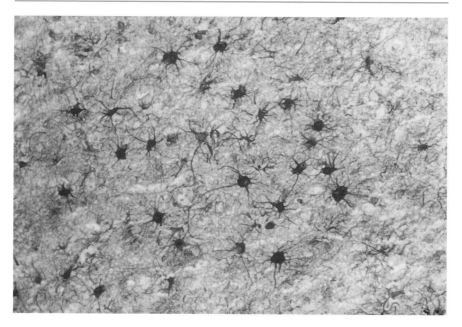

Figure 3 **Astrocytes** Star-shaped astrocytes in white matter near an acute plaque. Immunocytochemical staining with anti-glial fibrillary acidic protein antibody, magnification ×220. *(Courtesy of Dr J Newcombe, Institute of Neurology, London.)*

presumed to be largely due to loss of myelin and axons secondary to inflammatory damage.[81,82] Studies have shown that neurological disability correlates with spinal cord area or volume,[81,83,84] atrophy of infratentorial structures[84,85] and increased intracranial cerebrospinal fluid space.[86] Atrophy occurs early in the disease course[87] and is significantly influenced by inflammatory disease activity on MRI[87–89] and relapse rates.[90] Because anti-inflammatory therapy reduces the rate of brain atrophy in RR,[91] but not SP MS,[92] the importance of oedema to overall brain volume has been raised.

Attack   see *Relapse*.

Attack rate   number of attacks (relapses, exacerbations) in a given period, usually per annum. This varies with definition and the population under study. The rates are higher in younger patients and lower with longer disease duration.[298] Attacks are more frequent in the early years of RR MS (about 1–2 attacks per year on average, but varying widely from 0 to 12 or more) and significantly lower in patients with SP MS. The early attack rate is a negative prognostic factor for the rate and level of disability that will accumulate over subsequent decades (i.e. the higher the attack rate, the shorter the time to EDSS 6).[553] The effect of treatments on relapse rate is a frequent outcome measure in therapeutic trials and the natural decline of these events needs to be taken into account in the trial design, analysis and interpretation of results.

Autoantibody antibody against self- (auto)antigen.

Autoantigen self-antigen, antigen inducing an autoimmune response [see also *Autoimmune disease*].

Autoimmune disease pathological form of autoimmunity that results from the failure of the immune system to distinguish foreign proteins from normal tissue components (self vs non-self) resulting in damage to normal tissues. There is increasing evidence that MS has autoimmune pathological mechanisms. This includes female dominance (as seen in most autoimmune diseases), similarities to EAE, association with certain HLA antigens, association with other autoimmune diseases for patients or relatives, response to immunosuppressive or immunomodulatory drugs.

Autoimmunity immune response against antigens present in self-tissue or self-components. This may have pathological consequences (autoimmune disease), but also may be naturally occurring and even protective.

Avonex® (Biogen) see *Interferon beta-1a*.

Axon long fibre-like process of a nerve cell that is bundled together with many thousands of other axons to form the anatomical structure of a nerve and to conduct nerve impulses from the nerve cell body. [See *Figure 4*.] Axonal damage and transection occur in areas of active demyelination and inflammation and are likely to play a critical role in the development of irreversible deficits in MS.[93,94] There is increasing MRI evidence of axonal loss in lesions on magnetic transfer imaging,[95,96] diffusion tensor imaging[97] and magnetic spectroscopy.[98,99] Furthermore, axonal density correlates with the degree of spinal cord atrophy and volume of the normal appearing white matter.[100,101] [See also *Atrophy*.]

Azathioprine (Imuran) purine antimetabolite immunosuppressive agent that is relatively T-cell specific. Meta-analyses show that azathioprine reduces relapse rate after two years of treatment (*Table 4*) and slows disability after two to three years.[102] However, because of problems associated with the

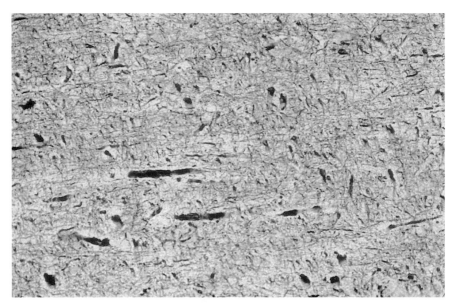

(A)

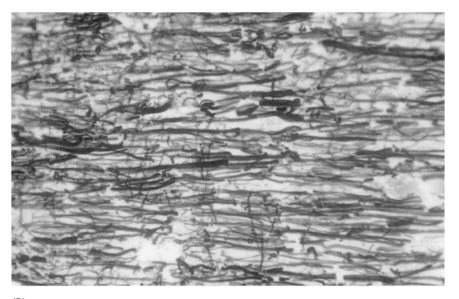

(B)

Figure 4 **Axons** A: A range of axon diameters in normal control brain white matter. B: Marked loss of axons, especially axons with fine diameters, and increased numbers of large-diameter axons, within an acute MS plaque. Immunocytochemical staining with anti-neurofilament antibody, magnification ×440. *(Courtesy of Dr J. Newcombe, Institute of Neurology, London.)*

16

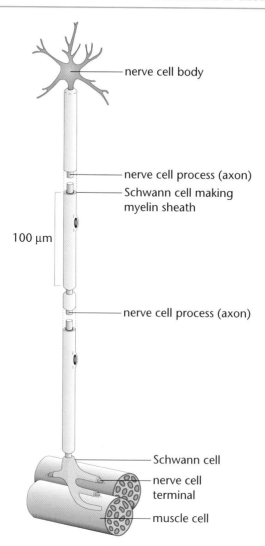

(C)

Figure 4 *(cont.)* C: Schematic representation of an axon in the peripheral nervous system, with its associated Schwann cells, contacting a muscle cell at a neuromuscular junction. Reproduced with permission.[21A]

Table 4 Effect of azathioprine on relapse rate

Reference	Reduction of relapse rate (%)	P value (years)	Study length	Type of MS
106[a]	−45	0.08	2	RR
107	−27	0.025	4	RR, SP
108	−50	0.02	3	SP
109	[b]Aza 0.92–0.79 Plac 0.6–0.67	NS	3	RR, SP
110[c]	−49	NS	2	RR

[a]Year 1, $P = 0.16$; year 2, $P = 0.05$.
[b]Pre- and post-treatment relapse rate.
[c]$n = 19$, azathioprine; $n = 24$, placebo; not intention to treat analysis.
Adapted with permission.[842]

nature and interpretation of meta-analyses, such data cannot be equated with Class I evidence from randomized placebo-controlled trials. No placebo-controlled studies of the effects of azathioprine on MRI have been performed so that its effects on disease burden and new lesion accumulation are unknown. The possible mechanism(s) underlying the effects of azathioprine include a reduction in the inflammatory response,[103] a decrease in the function of natural killer cells[104] and a decrease in antibody production.[105] Its side-effects include leukopenia, anorexia, abnormal liver function and possible increase in the risk of malignancy. Azathioprine is metabolized in part by S-methylation, which is catalysed by the enzyme thiopurine S-methyltransferase (TPMT). Three distinct groups of subjects can be identified by the activity of the level of TPMT in their red cells, which is inherited as a codominant trait. Individuals homozygous for low levels of TPMT activity have greatly elevated concentrations of the active 6-thioguanine metabolites, which increases their risk of life-threatening myelosuppression. Azathioprine and 6-mercaptopurine should, therefore, be avoided in patients with low enzymatic activity. It is now standard practice to measure red cell TPMT activity and to identify patients with low activity in which the drug is contra-indicated. Because of the lack of class I evidence and adverse effects, its use can only be condoned as a third-line therapy in highly selected patients with frequent and disabling exacerbations and/or rapid progression, or in a situation where newer immunomodulatory agents based on class I evidence are not available.

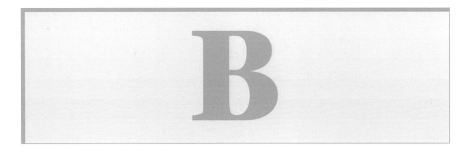

Bacille Calmette–Guerin (BCG) mycobacterial vaccines are potential immuno-modulatory agents.[111] In a single cross-over trial of 14 patients with RR MS, BCG vaccination significantly reduced MRI activity.[112] Further exploratory studies are planned.

Baclofen (Lioresal) structural analogue of GABA, one of the main inhibitory transmitters in the CNS. It is the most widely used antispastic agent in MS and several studies have demonstrated its efficacy.[113] Treatment is usually initiated with low daily doses (5 mg) to avoid adverse events, and increased in 5 mg increments at approximately 4–5-day intervals to a dose of 50–60 mg daily (or higher) in three or four divided doses. Side-effects include drowsiness, sedation and muscle weakness ('rag doll effect'). Intrathecal baclofen is also effective in reducing spasticity in MS, but this treatment is expensive, invasive and prone to complications. It is reserved for patients with severe refractory spasticity.[114] Baclofen has been shown to be as effective as, or more effective than, diazepam, but causes less sedation.[115,116]

Balo's concentric sclerosis rare form of MS in which the distinguishing pathological features are alternating bands of destruction and preservation of myelin in a series of concentric rings. Large plaques in the white matter are frequently distributed symmetrically in the cerebral hemispheres and cerebellum. It has been considered a variety of Schilder's disease, which it resembles in its clinical aspects and in the general distribution of lesions. Survival is generally under one year and the shortest published course two weeks.[117]

Barkhof diagnostic criteria see *MRI diagnostic criteria (of Barkhof)*.

Barthel Index measure of disability as independence in ten activities of daily living.[119] Items are rated from behavioural observation on a two-point (two items), three-point (six items) or four-point (two items) response scale and summed to generate a total score (low score indicates high disability).[120] It is used in stroke rehabilitation[54] and has been shown to be reliable, valid and responsive.[119,121]

B cells   see *B lymphocytes*.

Beck Depression Inventory   method of screening depression in medically ill patients.[122] It has a sensitivity of 71% and specificity of 79% in screening for major depression in early MS.[123]

Behçet's disease   rare, chronic, idiopathic, multisystem, inflammatory disorder with a relapsing–remitting clinical course. Cardinal features are recurrent oral and genital ulceration, and intraocular inflammation. Clinical involvement of the nervous system is reported in 4–49% of cases and most commonly consists of acute or subacute brain stem syndromes, cord lesions, aseptic meningitis, encephalitis and cerebral venous thrombosis. The mucocutaneous lesions and systemic manifestations (headache, fever, meningeal irritation and raised ESR) in acute attacks are usually diagnostic, but combinations of cranial nerve lesions, myelopathy and MRI abnormalities may cause confusion with MS.[124,125] The MRI may be indistinguishable from that of MS, but the absence of confluent periventricular lesions and presence of basal ganglia involvement may provide useful diagnostic clues.[126]

Benign MS   RR MS in which accumulated disability after a long period (usually in the range of 10–20 years) is either non-existent or mild. There is no agreed disability level or duration of observation required. A recent definition is that 'the patient remains fully functional in all neurologic systems 15 years after disease onset'.[127] Although the MRI is characterized by low levels of inflammatory activity, a high 'Burden of Disease' (BOD) may be present due to the long disease course prior to investigation. A 'diagnosis' of benign MS is retrospective and does not predict the future disease course. Follow-up studies show that most patients with this label eventually enter a disabling secondary progressive phase. On this basis the term 'benign MS' is potentially misleading. A more appropriate term for this category would be 'slow MS'.

Beta₂-microglobulin   biological marker of disease activity in autoimmune diseases that is actively secreted by lymphocytes.[128] It may provide a marker of lymphocyte activation within CSF.[129]

Betaferon, Betaseron   see *Interferon beta-1b*.

Black holes   qualitative term used to describe hypointense lesions in the white matter on T_1-weighted images (short TR/short TE spin echo image) [see *Figure 5*]. Acute black holes represent areas of oedema related to acute inflammation, whereas chronic black holes indicate persistent tissue destruction with expanded extracellular space and axonal loss.[130] Black hole measurements appear to be more specific for MS pathologies than T_2 total lesion load and correlate strongly with disability[131] and disease progression.[132] The development of T_1 black holes correlates with prior inflammatory disease activity and has been reduced by treatment with interferon β-1a in relapsing–remitting MS.[133] Black holes have been increasingly used as an MRI endpoint in phase III MS treatment trials.[133,134]

Bladder dysfunction   urinary symptoms are common in MS and have been estimated to occur in approximately 75% of all patients.[135,136] Bladder dysfunction is associated with the degree of pyramidal tract involvement and overall disability as measured by EDSS.[136-138] Urinary tract complications are a significant cause of morbidity in MS. Three basic patterns of dysfunction

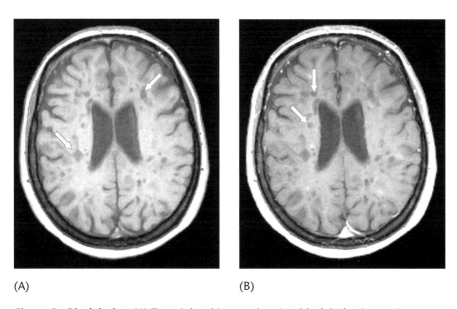

(A)   (B)

Figure 5   **Black holes** (A) T_1-weighted image showing black holes (arrows); (B) T_1-weighted image from the same patient following injection of gadolinium-DTPA. Note that some lesions enhance and others do not.

have been identified using urodynamics—detrusor hyper-reflexia, sphincter–detrusor dyssynergia and detrusor areflexia (see respective entries). The commonest symptoms, urgency, frequency and urge incontinence, correlate with detrusor hyper-reflexia,[136,137] and hesitancy of micturition with detrusor areflexia.[137] Bladder symptoms in MS patients should be evaluated by urodynamic studies prior to initiating treatment.

Bladder ultrasound　ultrasound examination of the bladder before and after micturition can establish the presence of incomplete emptying by estimated residual volume. Its advantages are that it is easy to perform, and is rapid and noninvasive. A residual volume of 100 ml or more is important for planning appropriate therapies.

Blood–brain barrier disruption, MRI　breakdown of the blood–brain barrier (BBB) is a consistent feature of new lesion development in relapsing–remitting and secondary progressive MS. T_1-weighted postgadolinium images are used to evaluate BBB integrity [see also *Gadolinium-enhancing lesion*]. Pathological studies show that areas of enhancement correlate with areas of active inflammation and macrophage-mediated myelin destruction.[139]

B lymphocytes (B cells)　cells that mediate the humoral immune response by producing soluble antibodies (immunoglobulins) that bind and prepare antigenic structures for phagocytosis or lysis (via complement cascade) and eventual elimination from the organism. Terminally differentiated B cells that produce antibodies are termed plasma cells. B cells also function as antigen presenting cells and produce cytokines [see also *Antibody, Humoral immune response* and *Immunoglobulin*].

Bone marrow transplantation　aggressive form of immune therapy used in treating MS. Although it appears to stop relapses and stabilize disease activity on MRI, it is not known whether it improves clinical outcome. It is poorly tolerated by patients with significant disability, has a high incidence of serious adverse effects[140] and is unlikely to be widely used.

Botulinum (BTX)　powerful toxin produced by the organism *Clostridium botulinum* which has been found to be useful in the treatment of an increasing range of conditions such as strabismus, blepharospasm, hemifacial spasm, focal dystonias and spasticity. It acts at the neuromuscular junction by inhibiting the release of acetylcholine. Several studies have reported efficacy in reducing spasticity.[141-143] BTX is widely used in MS, particularly for patients in the latter stages of progressive disease having problems with mobility, posture, continence and pain.

Bout   see *Relapse*.

Bowel function   constipation is the most commonly encountered symptom in MS populations, but up to 50% may also report faecal incontinence,[144,145] with or without urgency.

Box and Block Test   scale for upper extremity functional assessment in MS along with *Nine-Hole Peg Test*.[146]

Brainstem auditory evoked potential (BAEP)   series of electrical potentials produced by the brain and acoustic nerve in response to auditory stimulation (usually a monaural click). The major, clinically useful potentials include waves I and II that originate from the eighth nerve external to the brainstem, wave III from the cochlear nucleus, and waves IV and V from the regions bilaterally around the lateral lemniscus. Typical abnormalities found in MS patients include: prolongation of waves II–V, measured by the I–V interpeak latency; prolongation of I–II and III–V interpeak latencies; loss of amplitude of wave V, measured by V/I amplitude ratio; and disappearance of wave V.[147] Abnormalities of the BAEP are rather less frequent in clinically definite and suspected MS than the VEP or SEP,[148] but have been reported to be more sensitive than MRI for detecting pontine lesions.[149,150]

Brainstem syndrome, isolated   see *Isolated brainstem syndrome*.

The Brief Repeatable Battery   neuropsychological test battery developed by selecting the five tests that appear to be most sensitive to impairment in MS.[791] It consists of the Selective Reminding Test, the 10/36 Spatial Recall Test, the Symbol Digit Modalities Test, the Paced Auditory Serial Addition Test [see *Appendix 4*] and the Word List Generation Test. It is reported to be sufficiently brief to be used as a screening test with a sensitivity of 71% and a specificity of 94%.[204]

Burden of disease (BOD)   total estimated area in mm^2 or volume in mm^3 of hyperintense lesions identified on PD/T_2-MRI scans [see also *Total lesion load*].

Cambridge Basic Multiple Sclerosis Score (CAMS)   ordinal scale that rates the individual contributions of disability, relapse, disease progression and handicap by using four separate subscales with a five-level scoring system.[151] This scale is considered reproducible, responsive to relapse and progression domains, and highly correlated with FIM, EDSS and SNRS.[31,151] It was not designed as an outcome measure for clinical trials, or as a substitute for existing scales, but as a useful shorthand record for clinical neurological practice and retrospective case note analysis.[152]

Campath 1H (anti-CD52)   humanized monoclonal antibody against CD52, a pan-leukocyte marker with profound cytolytic properties resulting in prolonged leukocyte depletion. Use in MS may result in an acute transient worsening of current symptoms, or renewal of previous symptoms, associated with an increase in circulating levels of TNF-α, IL-6 and IFN-γ.[153,154] Campath 1H suppressed disease activity on MRI, but half the patients on treatment became progressively more disabled over time and MR studies showed progressive cerebral atrophy in those patients.[154,155] In addition, about 40% of patients on the treatment developed autoimmune thyroid disease in the second year of treatment

Candidate gene   gene whose product has been implicated in the cause of a disease either by location to an area of linkage, or by its known role in a pathway thought to be involved in pathogenesis.

Cannabis (tetrahydrocannabinol, marihuana)   has been considered an effective treatment for spasticity and tremor.[156,157] A double-blind, placebo-controlled, cross-over clinical trial in MS patients has demonstrated efficacy on spasticity.[158] Another study suggested some effect on action tremor.[159] However, in an exploratory phase II trial, treatment with either THC or plant-extract worsened the participant's global impression.[160] A large phase

III clinical trial in the UK will evaluate the efficacy of oral cannabinoids in reducing spasticity.

Carbamazepine membrane-stabilizing anti-epileptic drug that can be a highly effective treatment for many paroxysmal symptoms in MS, including trigeminal neuralgia.[161] It may also have some effects on postural and movement-induced tremor.[162]

Case fatality ratio proportion of affected subjects who die from a disease.

CD cluster of differentiation surface marker molecules on cells of the immune system.

CD1 expressed on APC (dendritic cells); involved in presentation of glycolipid antigens.

CD2 found on T cells; T cell adhesion molecule, involved in T cell activation.

CD3 found on (most) T cells (pan-T cell marker), involved in TCR signal transduction.

CD4 (T4 antigen) 56-kDa monomeric membrane glycoprotein that contains four extracellular immunoglobulin-like domains (D_1–D_4). It is present on approximately two-thirds of circulating human T cells. The antigen binds to the β_2-domain of class II MHC molecules on the APC and increases the avidity of the interaction between a T-cell receptor and a peptide–MHC complex.[163] [See also *CD4$^+$ T cells*.]

CD4$^+$ T cells cells expressing CD4$^+$ that are activated only by antigenic peptides complexed with MHC class II molecules (i.e. MHC class II restricted).[164] Class II MHC-restricted CD4$^+$ T cells produce cytokines and are associated with delayed-type hypersensitivity and antibody responses [see also *T-helper 1 cells* and *T-helper 2 cells*]. CD4$^+$ T cells are the key effectors in EAE. CD4$^+$ T cells are the primary cell type in the inflammatory infiltrates in MS lesions. Treatment with monoclonal anti-CD4 antibodies prevents the onset of EAE.[165,166] CD4$^+$ T cells can be classified into distinct populations—Th1 and Th2—on the basis of their patterns of cytokine production[167] [see also *T-helper 1 cells* and *T-helper 2 cells*]. Treatment of MS with anti-CD4 antibodies has not significantly suppressed the disease.[45,168,169] [See also *Anti-CD4*.]

CD4⁺/CD8⁺ cell ratio approximately 2 : 1 in normal human peripheral blood. May be significantly increased in MS, due primarily to a decrease in CD8⁺ T cells.[170]

CD5 found on B cell subsets (associated with polyreactivity) and some T cells.

CD8 (T8 antigen) membrane glycoprotein that contains α and β chains consisting of a single extracellular immunoglobulin-like domain, a hydrophobic transmembrane region, and a cytoplasmic tail containing 25–27 residues.[163] CD8 binds to the α3 domain of MHC class I and increases the avidity of the interaction between the T cell receptor and a peptide–MHC complex.[163] [See also *CD8⁺ T cells*.]

CD8⁺ T cells cells that express CD8 and generally function as cytotoxic (Tc) cells; they are bound and activated only by antigenic peptides complexed with MHC class I molecules (i.e. MHC class I restricted).[163] The role of CD8⁺ T cells in modulating the course of demyelinating disease is unclear, although CD8⁺ T cells may be predominant in many active demyelinating lesions.[171] The exact role of CD4⁺ and CD8⁺ T cells in human MS remains unresolved.[172] A dichotomy of CD8 cells in terms of cytokine production similar to the Th1/Th2 dichotomy has been described; these cell subtypes have been termed Tc1 and Tc2. [See also *T-cytotoxic cells*.]

CD11 a,b,c,d adhesion molecules.

CD11/CD18 integrin family that is involved in mediating immune cell migration into the CNS in inflammatory diseases [see also *Integrin*]. Humanized anti-CD11/CD18 antibodies have proved to be effective in reducing brain lesions in EAE and have been studied in a phase I trial in MS.[48] [See also *Anti-CD11/CD18 antibodies*.]

CD18 associated with CD11 (a–d) adhesion molecules.

CD25 IL-2 receptor α-chain; on activated T and B cells; targeting suppresses EAE; increased in MS.

CD26 peptidase on activated T cells; targeting suppresses EAE; increased in MS.

CD28   activation and costimulatory molecule on T cells.

CD40   found on APCs; involved in T cell–APC interaction via CD154 on activated T cells.

CD44   activation molecule on lymphocytes and leukocytes; adhesion molecule; interacts with hyaluronic acid; targeting suppresses EAE.

CD52   small surface protein on T and B cells. [See also *Campath 1H*.]

CD80 (B7.1)   costimulatory molecule on APCs; interacts with CD28, CTLA-4 (CD152); involved in EAE and MS.

CD86 (B7.2)   costimulatory molecule on APCs; interacts with CD28, CTLA-4 (CD152); involved in EAE and MS.

CD95 (Fas, Apo-1)   found on activated T, B and NK cells; induces apoptosis by interaction with ligand FasL; involved in EAE and MS.

CD152 (CTLA-4)   found on activated T cells and involved in negative regulation of T cell activation and costimulation; involved in EAE and MS.

CD154 (CD40L)   found on activated T cells; induces class switching and B cell proliferation by interacting with CD40 on B cells; cytokine production and activation in macrophages and other APC by interacting with CD40; increased in MS; blockade of the interaction suppresses EAE.

Cell adhesion molecules   see *Adhesion molecules*.

Central conduction time (CCT)   an estimate of the transit time of the ascending volley in the central segments of the somatosensory pathways. For median nerve stimulation, the measurement of the interpeak interval between the cervical N13 wave and the parietal N20 component is the most widely used in clinical practice. Prolongation of CCT has been considered to be a more sensitive measure than SEP response latencies.[173] [See also *Somatosensory evoked potential*.]

Central motor conduction time (CMCT)   an estimate of the transit time of the descending volley in the central segment of the motor pathways. It is measured as the difference between the cortical and spinal latency of motor evoked potentials (MEPs) (i.e. eliminates effects of peripheral motor pathway). Studies in MS have demonstrated marked prolongation of CMCT.[174-176] [See also *Magnetic evoked motor potential* and *Motor evoked potential*.]

Central scotoma   visual defect occupying the centre of the visual field. Optic neuritis has a predilection for the papillomacular fibres so that central or paracentral scotomata are commonly found in patients with MS. [See also *Visual field defect.*]

Cerebrospinal fluid (CSF)   fluid in the subarachnoid space surrounding the brain and spinal cord. Routine laboratory testing includes the total protein (usually less than 40 mg%), glucose $\frac{2}{3}$ or more of the simultaneous blood glucose level, white cells (no polymorphonuclear leucocytes and <5 lymphocytes) and immunoglobulins (no oligoclonal bands and normal IgG/albumin ratio).

Cervical spondylotic myelopathy (CSM)   degenerative disease of the spine (osteoarthritis), usually of the lower cervical vertebrae, that may narrow the spinal canal and intervertebral foramina and cause progressive damage to the spinal cord, roots, or both (particularly in individuals with constitutionally narrow cervical canals or predisposing occupations). In the absence of radicular signs and symptoms, the resulting spastic paraparesis may be clinically indistinguishable from spinal MS. MS and CSM may be significantly associated.[177] Radicular signs and symptoms (i.e. pain in segmental distribution, loss of reflexes, and segmental motor wasting and weakness) are sufficiently unusual in MS, particularly early on in the disease course, to indicate the need for investigation.

CHAMPS (Avonex®, Biogen)   phase III treatment trial that investigated the effect of weekly intramuscular injections of 30 μg of interferon β-1a for three years on 383 patients who had a first acute clinical demyelinating event.[178] The cumulative probability of developing CD MS was significantly lower in the interferon-treated group (35%) than in the placebo group (50%). The median increase in BOD was 1% in the interferon-treated group as compared with 16% in the placebo group and there were also fewer new/enlarging and gadolinium-enhancing lesions in the actively treated group than in the group on placebo.

Charcot variant   see *Chronic MS pathology.*

2-chlorodeoxyadenosine   see *Cladribine.*

Chemokines   small cytokines of relatively low molecular weight involved in the activation and migration of phagocytic cells and lymphocytes. The brain has been shown to express receptors for several chemokines and they are increasingly recognized as having a major role in inflammatory processes, including MS. Some chemokine receptors are also implicated as receptors for the HIV virus.

Chronic active plaque (of MS)   abnormal areas of white matter that have features of both the established chronic plaque and the acute MS lesion. Common features include zones of active inflammatory demyelination (often at the circumference of the plaque) with inflammatory cellular infiltrates and foamy macrophages actively removing and digesting myelin. Oligodendroglial cells are much reduced in number, axons may appear to be relatively preserved, but damaged, and there may be ongoing remyelination and hypertrophic astrocytes.[10,179] [See *Figure 6.*]

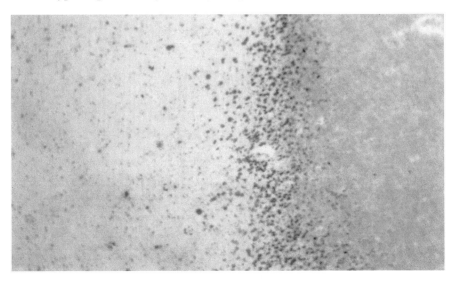

Figure 6 **Chronic active plaque** Myelin-filled macrophages (centre) at the actively demyelinating circumference of a chronic active plaque, with only scattered macrophages remaining in the demyelinated plaque on the left of the border, and macroscopically normal white matter on the right of the border. Oil red O and haematoxylin staining, magnification ×44. For full-colour version, please see accompanying CD. *(Courtesy of Dr J Newcombe, Institute of Neurology, London.)*

Chronic MS pathology (Charcot variant) the pathology of long-standing (usually chronically progressive) cases is characterized by the presence of multiple, sharply demarcated lesions of variable size, irregular shape and apparently random distribution, although with some propensity for the white matter abutting the surface of the lateral ventricles.[180] Macroscopically, lesions of different ages are usually present: acute plaques are pink due to hyperaemia associated with ongoing inflammation, or white to yellowish due to lipid breakdown and neutral fat production; chronic plaques are retracted or shrunken, grey–tan in colour and of firm consistency due to established gliosis. [See *Figure 7*.]

Chronic plaque (of MS) established lesion of the white matter that is predominantly a quiescent glial scar. There is often a sharply defined margin and abrupt transition to the surrounding normal myelin. The centre of a chronic plaque is commonly characterized by astroglial scar tissue, reduced numbers and diameter of axons,[96,181] depletion of oligodendrocytes[182–184] and sparse myelin staining.[10,179]

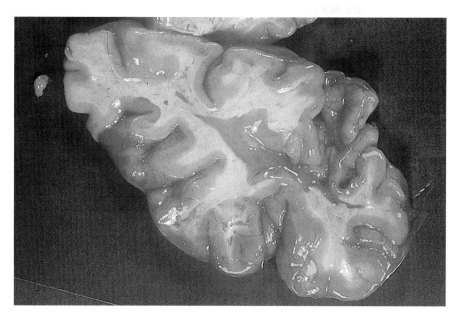

Figure 7 **Chronic MS pathology (Charcot variant):** Unfixed brain slice from a patient with MS showing a sharply demarcated large chronic inactive plaque on the wall of the ventricle, and small actively demyelinating plaques scattered through the white matter. For full-colour version, please see accompanying CD. *(Courtesy of Dr J Newcombe, Institute of Neurology, London.)*

Cladribine (2-chlorodeoxyadenosine, 2-CdA) highly specific antilympho-
cyte agent that results in lymphocyte death by apoptosis.[185] In a phase II
study, patients with 'progressive MS' treated with cladribine showed an
improvement in SNRS scores and a decrease in new or active lesions on
MRI.[186] In a subsequent phase III study of PP and SP MS, no clinical benefits
(on EDSS or SNRS) were found, despite a significant positive effect on
MRI activity.[187] Cladribine was well tolerated, with the exception of a dose-
dependent lymphocytopenia and thrombocytopenia. In the absence of a
convincing effect on sustained progression of disability, it is unlikely that
cladribine will be widely accepted or used as an alternative disease-
modifying therapy for patients with SP MS.[188] Trials of cladribine in RR MS
are currently being considered.

Classification (diagnostic) of MS see *Diagnostic criteria, clinical*.

Classification of disease course see *Disease course, classification*.

Clinically definite MS (CD MS) category in the Poser Committee criteria in
which two clinical 'attacks' or relapses and clinical evidence of two separate
lesions; or two attacks with clinical evidence of one lesion and paraclinical
evidence of another separate lesion, are required for a clinically definite diagnosis [see *Table 9*].[191] The two attacks must involve different parts of the
CNS, must be separated by a period of at least a month and each must last a
minimum of 24 hours. The term 'clinically definite' is not recommended in
the latest diagnostic criteria.[192]

Clinically isolated syndrome the most common clinical presentation of MS
is a young adult with acute or subacute optic neuritis, myelopathy or a
brainstem syndrome, i.e. a symptom complex that is related to a single site
in the nervous system ('clinically isolated') with no clinical evidence of multiple lesions in space and time. The risk of developing further attacks and
thus 'clinically definite' MS[13–15,197,198] depends on the demonstration of other
'clinically silent' lesions by investigations with MRI or evoked potentials.[14,199]
[See also *Acute (subacute) myelopathy, Isolated brainstem syndrome* and *Optic
neuritis*.]

Clinically probable MS (CP MS) diagnostic category in the Poser Committee
criteria[191] that requires: (i) two attacks and clinical evidence of one lesion,
(ii) one attack and clinical evidence of two separate lesions, (iii) one attack,

clinical evidence of one lesion and paraclinical evidence of another, separate lesion. [See *Table 9*.] The category 'probable MS' is not recommended in the latest scheme.[192]

Cluster   an apparent excess of cases of a disease that occurs within a small geographical area. Cluster analysis is a potentially powerful strategy for revealing the aetiology of a disease,[200] but many apparent clusters can be attributed to chance or to altered recognition and shifts in diagnostic procedures.[201] Two types of cluster analysis are *Post hoc* and *Space–time*.

Cognitive dysfunction   cognitive impairment in MS resembles the pattern seen in subcortical dementias [see also *Subcortical dementia*]. Between 55% and 65% of patients with MS are thought to have some cognitive impairment, which is more frequent and severe in patients with the chronic-progressive form of disease.[202-206] Deficits of anterograde memory,[207] difficulties with tasks that require rapid information processing[207,208] and problem solving,[209-211] or mood disturbances[203,212] are commonly reported in patients with MS, and may contribute to cognitive impairment. The presumed mechanism underlying subcortical dementia is disconnection of pathways linking subcortical structures with cortical areas or the limbic cortex.[211] No relationship between degree of cognitive disturbance and degree of disability has been found.[205-207] Total lesion area appears the best MRI predictor of deficits of recent memory, whereas size of corpus callosum predicts deficits in information-processing speed.[211]

Cold   cooling by air conditioning or swimming enables some fibres, which are blocked at normal body temperature, to conduct, with a consequent improvement in symptoms and function in some temperature-sensitive patients.

Colour vision   see *Dyschromatopsia*.

Combined unique active lesions (CU active lesions)   MRI measure of disease activity on serial images that avoids double counting of lesions showing simultaneous T_2 and T_1 activities. When a T_1-enhancing lesion and a T_2 active lesion are determined to be the same lesion, the lesion is linked. Links can involve the current, previous or subsequent scan in the series. Non-linked T_1-enhancing lesions and non-linked PD/ T_2 active lesions and the linked lesions are then combined to give counts of new combined unique active lesions.[213] CU active lesions have been used as a primary outcome for phase III clinical trials.[213] The median number of CU active lesions was reduced by 80.7% (22 μg) and 87.5% (44 μg) for MS patients treated with interferon-β1a.[213]

Complement (C) major effector of the humoral branch of the immune system that consists of 20 soluble plasma and body fluid proteins, together with cellular receptors on blood and tissue cells. Activated by three mechanisms, all converging at C3: a classical pathway via antigen–antibody complexes, an alternative pathway involving the direct activation of C3 and the lectin pathway where carbohydrate residues activate the mannose-binding lectin which, in turn, activates complement. Complement components interact to generate reaction products that facilitate antigen clearance and generation of an inflammatory response after an initial antigen–antibody reaction.[163] Complement is implicated as an amplifier of inflammatory processes. CSF studies provide evidence for complement activation in MS.[214–217] However, recent evidence shows that C3-deficient mice remain susceptible to EAE.[218]

Concentric plaque of Balo lesion characterized by concentric alternating layers of myelinated and demyelinated areas seen in some acute or rapidly progressive variants. The rings can sometimes be detected on MRI.[219]

Concordance twin pair in which both members exhibit the same phenotype or trait. Two separate and independent population-based twin studies performed in Canada[220] have identified concordance rates of 25–30% for MS in monozygotic twins, compared with 4.7% in dizygotic twins.

Conduction block failure of generation of an action potential at the nodes of Ranvier due to the loss of myelin in the paranodal region may result in slowing or failure of conduction through a nerve segment.[221] Weakness, numbness and other 'negative' symptoms of MS can be attributed either to blocked conduction or to critical loss of axons in a pathway.

Confirmed progression endpoint widely used in therapeutic clinical trials to measure deterioration in disability. It has been defined as an increase in the EDSS over baseline that is recorded or confirmed on at least two consecutive examinations at scheduled visits in a trial.[222] It was initially proposed as a method to recruit SP MS patients with aggressive disease for clinical trials,[223] and was thought to be more stable than the unconfirmed progression end-point.[224] Since then it has been 'borrowed' for RR MS trials where it is arguably less appropriate. The definition can have varying degrees of stringency, for example, the increase in disability required could be 1 or 2 points on the EDSS and the period between the two examinations could be 3, 6, 9 or 12 months. Most trials have used a 1.0 increase of EDSS confirmed on two occasions 3 or 6 months apart, but it is not always clear whether improvement between the two qualifying assessments is allowed (e.g. if monthly assessments showed the EDSS increase was not sustained). Studies of placebo patients show that this endpoint is unreliable for patients with RR MS as an increase in disability frequently reverts to baseline (i.e. is erroneous).[225] For this reason some patients may experience several so-called 'confirmed progressions'. Similarly, increasing the stringency of the definition does not necessarily increase the predictive accuracy for persistent disability.[225]

Construct validity   process used to establish the validity of a measurement instrument when no criterion (gold standard), or universe of content, is accepted as entirely adequate to define the attribute being measured.[226] It is used to examine the validity of clinical scales in MS and to evaluate their ability to detect differences in disability between groups and individuals. It is assessed using Pearson's and Spearman's rank correlation coefficients for interval and ordinal scales, respectively.

Contrast sensitivity   relative sensitivity of visual function to a visual stimulus at different levels of contrast. After optic neuritis, visual acuity measured on a high contrast Snellen card may be restored to normal or near-normal levels, i.e. 20/20 to 20/30. However, the frequent residual symptoms are due to preferential damage to channels carrying low-contrast visual information.[227,228] More than 50% of patients with normal visual acuity after optic neuritis may have demonstrable abnormalities of contrast sensitivity.[229]

Copaxone (Copolymer 1)   see *Glatiramer acetate*.

Core battery   neuropsychological research battery that provides a global dementia screen.[230] It consists of six cognitive domains including general knowledge,[231] attention–concentration,[232,233] memory,[234,235] language,[236,237] visuo-spatial functions[231] and abstract/conceptual reasoning.[231,238] The coverage of the battery is broad, but several tests are insensitive, impractical and/or poorly suited to longitudinal studies. For these reasons, the core battery has been considered unsuitable for MS research.[239]

Corpus callosum (CC)   largest white matter tract connecting the two cerebral hemispheres that plays an important role in the performance of complex tasks requiring precise timing of information transfer between multiple brain regions. CC atrophy is common in MS and correlates with cognitive impairment and,[211,242,243] reduced speed and accuracy on information processing tasks.[243] The CC is a common site for MS pathology with a reported prevalence of lesions between 2% and 55% on radiological evidence.[240,241] Abnormalities in the CC may be focal plaques or atrophy.[84,240] Hyperintensity on the undersurface of the CC (also termed the callosal–septal interface) on a midsagittal (long TR/short TE spin echo) image has been considered a relatively specific indicator of MS[241] [see *Table 22*]. The detection on FLAIR images of earlier, subtle findings, such as subcallosal striations, may be an aid to early diagnosis.[244] [See *Figure 8*.]

Cortical lesion   lesion situated primarily, or mainly, within the cortical grey matter. In contrast to periventricular lesions, cortical lesions are usually small—a few millimetres in diameter, or less [see *Figure 9*]. They may comprise between 26% and 30% of all lesions in MS[245] and a role in

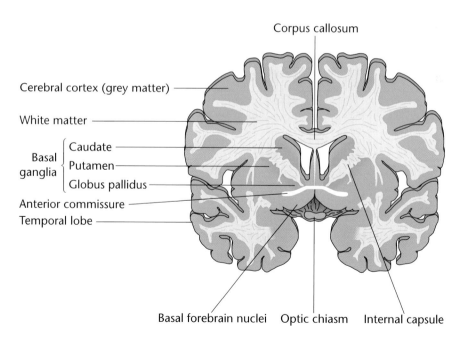

Figure 8   **Corpus callosum:** Internal structures of the brain as seen in coronal section (plane of section through the basal ganglia). Reproduced with permission.[843]

35

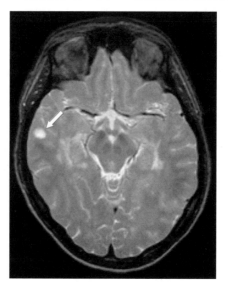

Figure 9 **Cortical lesion:** T_2-weighted image showing a cortical lesion (arrow) in clinically definite multiple sclerosis.

neuropsychological impairment has been suggested.[246,247] Fast FLAIR sequences appear to be sensitive to cortical lesions.[248-250] [See also *Fluid-attenuated inversion-recovery imaging*.]

Corticomedullary lesion   see *Juxtacortical lesion*.

Corticosteroids or glucocorticosteroids (steroids)   drugs with an established role in reducing the duration of relapses, particularly pulsed methylprednisolone, oral prednisolone or dexamethasone. They speed recovery from exacerbations and may, perhaps, reduce the risk of developing clinically definite MS in patients with a first episode of monosymptomatic optic neuritis.[251] Unfotunately, there is no evidence of any effect on the persistent disability or impairment resulting from an attack, i.e. the outcome of a relapse will be the same with or without steroid treatment. High-dose intravenous methylprednisolone 1 g daily for 3 days has become the preferred therapy for MS exacerbations, but recent studies have suggested that equivalent high oral doses may be equally effective.[252,253] Steroids in high doses have been shown to reduce gadolinium-enhanced lesions.[254-256] The mechanism(s) underlying these effects include reducing endothelium and capillary permeability,[257] decreasing lymphocyte proliferation and production of interferon-γ and tumour necrosis factor,[258] and inducing transforming growth factor β-1.[259] There is no established indication for the long-term use of these agents in view of side-effects and the lack of efficacy on natural history, e.g. relapse rates and disability accumulation.[260] [See also *Dexamethasone, Methylprednisolone and Prednisolone*.] The majority of steroid trials, however, were performed in the pre-MRI era when MS trials were not sufficiently powered.

Costimulation activation with acquisition of T cell effector function requires T cell activation via the trimolecular complex in combination with a 'second signal', the absence of which may lead to anergy. Costimulation involves interaction of surface molecules on T cells (other than the TCR) and APCs.

CSF/serum albumin quotient quotient of the average normal CSF albumin concentration divided by the average normal serum albumin concentration. Albumin is synthesized only in the liver, and is not catabolized within the CNS.[261] The absolute concentration of CSF albumin depends on many factors, including its blood concentration, BBB integrity, rate of CSF flow and age.[262] The CSF/serum quotient provides an assessment of the overall integrity of the BBB. An increased quotient is indicative of the excess albumin in the CSF that has crossed and damaged the BBB.[195]

Cumulative frequency see *Lifetime risk*.

Cyclophosphamide (Cytoxan®) antimitotic and immunosuppressive agent that suppresses T-helper cells and B lymphocytes, thus normalizing the ratio of T-helper to T-suppressor cells[263] and decreasing synthesis of IgG within the blood–brain barrier.[264,265] Although several unblinded trials of cyclophosphamide in chronic progressive MS have suggested a positive treatment effect,[29,266] these benefits have not been confirmed in placebo-controlled trials.[267,268] Because of the conflicting evidence for efficacy and serious adverse effects, including alopecia, haemorrhagic cystitis, leucopenia and malignancy, a role for cyclophosphamide in the treatment of MS has not been established.

Cyclosporine hydrophobic cyclic undecapeptide immunosuppressant. Clinical trials have suggested some benefits for patients with active relapsing–remitting or progressive MS.[269,270] Cyclosporine has not gained wide support because of severe adverse effects, particularly renal toxicity.[270]

37

Table 5 Sources and major effects of cytokines

Cytokine	Source	Effects on			
		B	T	M	OC
IL-1	M, OC	+	+	+	+ (pleiotropic effects on many cells)
IL-2	Th1, OC	+	+	+	+ (haematopoetic growth factor)
IL-3	T, OC			+	+ (pleiotropic effects on many cells)
IL-4	Th2, OC	+	+ (Th2)		+ (eosinophils)
IL-5	Th2, OC	+			
IL-6	Th2, B, M, OC	+	+		+ (release of acute phase proteins; haematopoetic factor)
IL-7	Stromal cells	+ (pre-B cells)	+ (thymocytes)		
IL-8	M, T, OC		+ (attractant)		+ (neutrophil attractant, angiogenic factor)
IL-9	T	+	+		+ (erythroid precursors)
IL-10	T, B, M, OC	+	+ (Th2), − (Th1)	−	+ or −(OC)
IL-11	Stromal cells				+ (haematopoetic progenitors)
IL-12	M, B, OC		+ (Th1)		+ (NK, haematopoetic cells)
IL-13	Th2	+		+ or −	
IL-14	B, T, OC	+			
IL-15	M, many OC	+			+ or −(OC)
IL-16	T (CD8)		+ (chemoattractant for CD4$^+$T)	++ (attractant for CD4$^+$M)	
IL-1 ra	M, OC	−	−	−	−(many OC)
IFN-α	B, T, M		Complex actions		
IFN-β	Fibroblasts, OC		Complex actions		
IFN-γ	T, OC		Complex actions		
TNF-α	M, T, OC	+	+	+	+ (pleiotropic effects on many cells)
LT	T, OC		Similar to TNF-α		
TGF-β	Many cells	−	−	+ or −	+ or − (highly pleiotropic, see text)

+ = stimulatory effect; − = inhibitory effect (blank = unknown, minor or absent effect); B = B lymphocyte; IFN = interferon; IL = interleukin; IL-1 ra = IL-1 receptor antagonist; LT = lymphotoxin; M = monocyte/macrophage; OC = other cells; T = T-lymphocyte; TGF = transforming growth factor; Th1 = T-helper-1 cells; TNF = tumour necrosis factor.
Adapted and modified with permission.[21]

Cytokines soluble glycoproteins secreted by immune system cells that modulate immune and inflammatory responses.[271] They are divided into two broad categories: pro- and anti-inflammatory cytokines. Pro-inflammatory cytokines, including tumour necrosis factor (TNF), interleukin 1 (IL-1), interleukin 2 (IL-2), and interferon gamma (IFN-γ), are associated with the T-helper type 1 (Th1) cell subclass, and upregulate cell mediated inflammatory responses. Anti-inflammatory cytokines include transforming growth factor beta (TGFβ), interferons alpha (IFNα) and beta (IFNβ) and interleukin-10 (IL-10). Interleukin 4 (IL-4), associated with the T-helper type 2 (Th2) subclass is involved in allergic inflammation, but downregulates cell-mediated immune responses. Cytokines play an important role in MS, based on studies of both the EAE animal model and human disease.[272] The pro-inflammatory cytokines are considered to induce or worsen disease features in MS. In contrast, anti-inflammatory cytokines are thought to be protective and to ameliorate disease features in MS [see *Table 5*].

Cytotoxic T cells see *T-cytotoxic cells*.

Cytoxan see *Cyclophosphamide*.

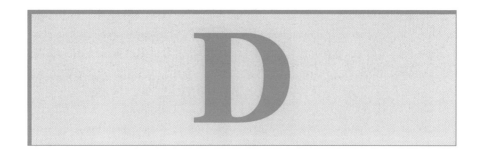

Dantrolene sodium hydantoin derivative that suppresses the release of calcium ions from the sarcoplasmic reticulum and has antispastic effects. Its use is limited by its side-effects, particularly hepatotoxicity.[273]

Dawson's finger eponym applied to the perivascular pattern of demyelination that resembles a 'finger' pointing along the course of a vessel.[274] The perivenous distribution of demyelination results in elongated lesions around periventricular vessels that run a course perpendicular to the ventricular wall. The ovoid hyperintense lesions radiating out from the ventricles on MRI are considered the radiological equivalent of Dawson's finger.[275] [See *Figure 10*.]

Dementia progressive deterioration of cognitive abilities in the absence of clouded consciousness [see also *Subcortical dementia*].

Demyelinating disease disease in which the pathological process primarily attacks the myelin sheaths of nerve fibres in the central and/or peripheral nervous systems. [See *Table 6*.]

Demyelination term applied to the pathological destruction of myelin sheaths around axons. 'Secondary demyelination' refers to the loss of myelin from nerve sheaths that follows axonal destruction in Wallerian degeneration. In the pathology, which has been thought to be predominant in MS, myelin sheaths are selectively destroyed and the axons at least partially preserved ('primary' demyelination). However, MS pathology also includes variable loss of oligodendrocytes and axonal transection and degeneration in areas of acute inflammation.[81] Current concepts of pathogenesis of MS include a T cell directed, macrophage-mediated myelinolytic process that results in areas of damaged myelin or 'plaques'.[172] [See *Figure 11*.]

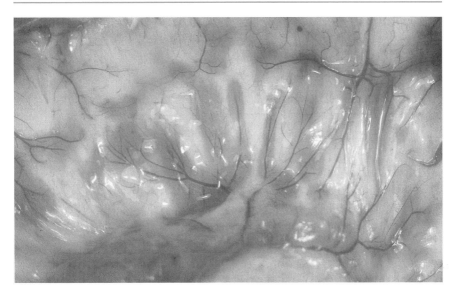

(A)

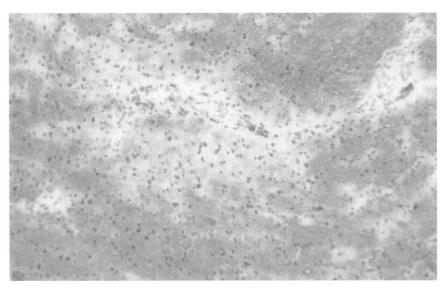

(B)

Figure 10 **Dawson's finger:** A: Unfixed brain slice with demyelinated areas running along veins which resemble "fingers" along the blood vessels running on the surface of the ventricular wall. B: Myelin loss along veins in brain white matter. Oil red O and haematoxylin staining, magnification ×110. For full-colour version, please see accompanying CD. *(Courtesy of Dr J Newcombe, Institute of Neurology, London.)*

Table 6 Classification of the demyelinating diseases. Some of these diseases are sometimes called dysmyelinating diseases because the pathology is defects in myelin production and maintenance rather than destruction of normal myelin

Isolated demyelinating syndromes
Acute haemorrhagic leucoencephalomyelitis—Hurst's disease
Acute disseminated encephalomyelitis
Optic neuritis
Cord lesions
    Acute necrotizing myelitis
    Transverse myelitis
    Chronic progressive myelopathy
    Radiation myelopathy
    HTLV-I associated myelopathy
Monophasic isolated demyelination—site unspecified

Multiple sclerosis
Relapsing-remitting
Secondary progressive
Primary progressive
Benign
Malignant or Marburg variant
Childhood
Silent multiple sclerosis
Devic's disease
Balo's concentric sclerosis
Combined central and peripheral demyelination

Central pontine myelinolysis
Pontine
Extrapontine

Diffuse sclerosis
Schilder's disease
    Myelinoclastic diffuse sclerosis
    Transitional diffuse sclerosis

Table 6 Continued.

Adrenoleucodystrophy

X-linked childhood adrenoleucodystrophy

X-linked adult-onset adrenomyeloneuronopathy

Autosomal recessive neonatal adrenoleucodystrophy

Autosomal recessive Zellweger's syndrome

Other leucodystrophies

Metachromatic leucodystrophy

    Late infantile

    Juvenile

    Adult

    Multiple sulphatase deficiency

Globoid cell

    Krabbe's disease

    Late-onset

    Canavan's disease

    Alexander's disease

Pelizaeus-Merbacher disease

    Connatal form

    Late-onset

    Other sudanophilic leucodystrophies

Depression prevalence rates for depression in patients with MS have been reported between 27% and 54%.[276,277] It is more common than euphoria. Depression has been variably attributed to a reaction to disability and poor health,[278] or directly to the disease process itself.[279,280] [See also *Suicide.*]

Destructive lesion term usually applied to severe and rapidly progressing acute and chronic MS lesions, in which demyelination is accompanied by extensive additional tissue destruction that may give rise to cystic brain lesions.[281] [See also *Black holes.*]

Detrusor areflexia inability to evoke a detrusor contraction when attempting to initiate voiding. In contrast to the universal finding of a high incidence of detrusor hyperreflexia, urodynamic studies have shown incidences of

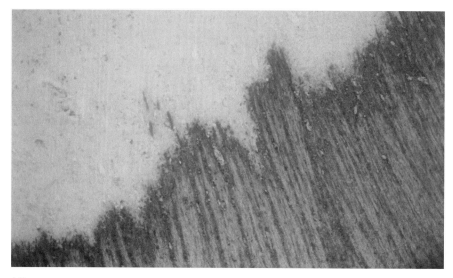

(A)

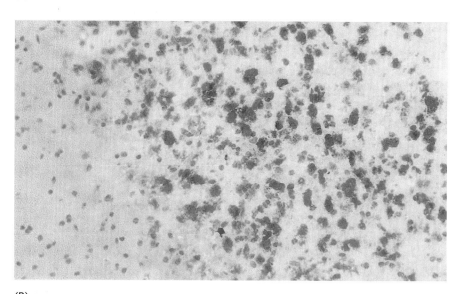

(B)

Figure 11 **Demyelination:** A: Myelin is completely lost from this MS plaque, with macroscopically normal myelinated white matter to the right. Immunocytochemical staining with an antibody directed against galactocerebroside, a myelin lipid. Magnification ×44. B: Macrophages containing degraded myelin lipids at the edge of a demyelinating plaque. Oil red O and haematoxylin staining. Magnification ×220. For full-colour version, please see accompanying CD. *(Courtesy of Dr J Newcombe, Institute of Neurology, London.)*

detrusor areflexia between 0% and 40% with or without hesitancy.[136,137,282-284] [See also *Urodynamics*.]

Detrusor hyperreflexia spontaneous detrusor contraction that the patient is unable to inhibit regardless of urinary volume (basically a failure to store urine). It is the commonest abnormality of detrusor function in MS with a frequency between 52% and 78%.[137,283,285] Detrusor hyperreflexia is commonly manifested symptomatically as urgency, frequency and generalized irritative symptoms.[136,137,286] It has been attributed to the interruption of the descending inhibitory pathway to the bladder regulatory centre in the lateral columns of the sacral cord.[137] [See also *Detrusor–sphincter dyssynergia* and *Urodynamics*.]

Detrusor–sphincter dyssynergia involuntary contraction of the external sphincter during a detrusor contraction that interrupts or prevents complete voiding. May be present in as many as 50% of patients.[284,287] Almost always associated with a suprasacral spinal cord lesion.[284] More than half of the patients with detrusor hyperreflexia also demonstrate detrusor–sphincter dyssynergia.[286,288] Clinical effects range from retention to total incontinence. Patients with detrusor hyperreflexia and appropriate sphincter relaxation are treated with anticholinergic agents, while patients who have detrusor hyperreflexia and detrusor–sphincter dyssynergia may be treated with anticholinergics and intermittent catheterization.[284,288]

Devic's neuromyelitis optica ('Devic's disease') demyelinating disease characterized by an acute–subacute onset of loss of vision in one or both eyes preceded or followed within days or weeks by a transverse or ascending myelitis.[289] Lesions in the spinal cord are extensive with isolated or confluent areas of tissue destruction. While the pathology of Devic's disease appears distinct from classical MS, individuals surviving the acute episode may subsequently develop a disease course typical of MS, suggesting that the underlying processes are similar or identical.[290] Features that are not characteristic of classical MS include a preponderance of non-Caucasians, a poor neurological recovery from relapses, a high frequency of normal brain MRI, a low frequency of CSF oligoclonal bands, unusually extensive spinal cord lesions and a high frequency of organ-specific autoantibodies.[291]

Dexamethasone oral steroid more powerful than prednisolone that has been used for treating relapses of MS. It is usually given in a tapering course of 2 to 3 weeks, or less.

45

Diagnosis (of MS)   usually made on clinical grounds through a careful history and neurological examination. A diagnosis of 'clinically definite MS' (CD MS)[190] or, on the new diagnostic schema,[192] 'MS' (which has replaced CD MS) can be made without the need for laboratory tests. In other patients with an unusual phenotype or obscure history, laboratory diagnostic tests, including MRI of the brain and/or spinal cord and lumbar puncture and blood tests, may be required to confirm dissemination of lesions in space and time and to exclude other conditions.

Diagnostic criteria, clinical (McDonald)   latest diagnostic scheme that integrates clinical, MRI and other paraclinical diagnostic methods.[192] The diagnostic outcomes are 'MS', 'possible MS' (for those at risk of MS, but with equivocal investigations) or 'not MS' (other neurological conditions). [See *Table 7*.]

Diagnostic criteria, clinical (McDonald and Halliday)   scheme for clinical diagnosis in which the demonstration of objective signs of lesions at two or more necessarily distinctive sites in the white matter is based either on physical examination or on electrophysiological tests.[190] [See *Table 8*.]

Diagnostic criteria, clinical (Poser)   criteria that incorporate historical and clinical symptomatology and paraclinical evidence, including results of cerebrospinal fluid examination (NB either presence of oligoclonal bands or raised IgG/albumin index is acceptable), neurophysiological tests and neuroimaging.[191] In this scheme, the proposed classification of MS comprises two major groups, definite and probable, each with two subgroups, clinical and laboratory-supported MS. Possible or latent MS is not included. [See *Table 9*.]

Diagnostic criteria, clinical (Schumacher)   diagnostic scheme based on natural history and physical findings.[189] The scheme was originally established in order to select patients for therapeutic trials. It defines 'clinically definite MS' without the inclusion of laboratory or paraclinical data. [See *Table 10*.]

Diagnostic criteria, MRI   see *MRI diagnostic criteria*.

Diagnostic 'red flags'   features sufficiently unusual and/or associated with a higher risk of misdiagnosis that should alert the neurologist to the possibility that a suggested or established 'diagnosis' of MS may be incorrect, or at least needs to be carefully reconsidered [see *Table 11*].

Table 7 McDonald Committee diagnostic criteria scheme

Clinical presentation	Additional data needed for MS diagnosis
Two or more attacks; objective clinical evidence of two or more lesions	None[a]
Two or more attacks; objective clinical evidence of one lesion	Dissemination in space, demonstrated by MRI[b] or two or more MRI-detected lesions consistent with MS plus positive CSF[c] or await further clinical attack implicating a different site
One attack; objective clinical evidence of two or more lesions	Dissemination in time, demonstrated by MRI[d] or second clinical attack
One attack; objective clinical evidence of one lesion (monosymptomatic presentation; clinically isolated syndrome)	Dissemination in space, demonstrated by MRI[b] or two or more MRI-detected lesions consistent with MS plus positive CSF[c] and dissemination in time, demonstrated by MRI[d] or second clinical attack
Insidious neurological progression suggestive of MS	Positive CSF[c] and dissemination in space, demonstrated by (a) 9 or more T_2 lesions in brain, or (b) two or more lesions in spinal cord, or (c), 4–8 brain plus one spinal cord lesion or abnormal VEP[e] associated with 4–8 brain lesions or, with fewer than 4 brain lesions plus one spinal cord lesion demonstrated by MRI and dissemination in time, demonstrated by MRI,[d] or continued progression for one year

If criteria indicated are fulfilled, the diagnosis is multiple sclerosis (MS); if the criteria are not completely met, the diagnosis is 'possible MS'; if the criteria are fully explored and not met, the diagnosis is 'not MS'.

[a] No additional tests are required; however, if tests [magnetic resonance imaging (MRI), cerebral spinal fluid (CSF)] are undertaken and are negative, extreme caution should be taken before making a diagnosis of MS. Alternative diagnoses must be considered. There must be no better explanation for the clinical picture.

[b] MRI demonstration of space dissemination must fulfil the criteria derived from Barkhof et al.[118] and Tintore et al.[193]

[c] Positive CSF determined by oligoclonal bands detected by established methods (preferably isoelectric focusing) different from any such bands in serum or by a raised IgG index.[194,195]

[d] MRI demonstration of time dissemination must fulfil the criteria listed in the table

[e] Abnormal visual evoked potential of the type seen in MS (delay with a well-preserved wave form).[196]

Reproduced with permission.[192]

47

Table 8 McDonald and Halliday's criteria for the classification of cases of multiple sclerosis

Classification	Criteria	Notes
Proved	Diagnosis established at necropsy	
Clinically definite	Remitting and relapsing history with two or more episodes and:	A relapse is reckoned as a period of at least 24 hours in which there is worsening of an existing symptom or group of symptoms, provided that the course has been stationary or has improved during the previous month[189]
	• evidence of lesions at two or more necessarily separate sites in the CNS and	Bilateral optic nerve lesions are counted as a single lesion only
	• lesions predominantly in the white matter and	
	• age at onset of symptoms 10–15 years and	
	• history of signs or symptoms for 1 year or longer and	Cases of shorter duration otherwise fulfilling these criteria are classed as 'early probable'
	• no better explanation for the observed abnormalities	

Early probable or latent	• Single episode suggestive of MS and • evidence of lesions at two or more necessarily separate sites in the CNS *or* • remitting and relapsing course and • evidence of only one lesion associated with MS	Cases suggestive of acute disseminated encephalomyelitis and transverse myelitis are excluded
Progressive probable	• Progressive history of paraplegia and • evidence of lesions at two or more necessarily separate sites in the CNS and • other causes excluded	
Progressive possible	• Progressive history of paraplegia and • evidence of only one lesion and • other causes excluded	
Suspected	• Single episode suggestive of MS without evidence of any lesion or with evidence of a single lesion only *or* • Recurrent optic neuritis (unilateral or bilateral) with one additional episode not involving the optic nerve but without evidence of lesions outside the eye	Recurrent optic neuritis without other features is excluded

Reproduced with permission.[190]

Table 9 Poser Committee clinical and laboratory diagnostic criteria for MS

Category	Attacks	Clinical evidence		Paraclinical evidence	CSF OB/IgG
Clinically definite					
CD MS 1	2	2			
CD MS 2	2	1	and	1	
Laboratory-supported definite					
LSD MS 1	2	1	or	1	+
LSD MS 2	1	2			+
LSD MS 3	1	1	and	1	+
Clinically probable					
CP MS 1	2	1			
CP MS 2	1	2			
CP MS 3	1	1	and	1	
Laboratory-supported probable					
LSP MS	2				+

CD MS = clinically definite MS; LSD MS = laboratory-supported definite MS;
CP MS = clinically probable MS; LSP MS = laboratory-supported probable MS;
OB/IgG = oligoclonal bands or increased IgG/albumin index in cerebrospinal fluid (CSF).

Reproduced with permission.[191]

Table 10 Schumacher's criteria for diagnosis of MS

- Neurologic examination reveals objective abnormalities of CNS function
- History indicates involvement of two or more parts of CNS
- CNS disease predominantly reflects white matter involvement
  - two or more episodes, each lasting at least 24 hours and $\geq$1 month apart
  - slow or stepwise progression of signs and symptoms over at least 6 months
- Patient 10–15 years old at onset
  Signs and symptoms cannot be better explained by other disease process

Reproduced with permission.[189]

Table 11 Diagnostic 'red flags'

- Symptoms and signs relating to a single site in the nervous system
- Positive family history of neurological disease (even 'MS')
- Signs suggesting a clear spinal level
- No signs or symptoms above the level of the foramen magnum
- Signs of lower motor neurone involvement (e.g. absent reflexes)
- Patients presenting at less than 15 or greater than 60 years of age
- Progressive disease from onset with no remissions
- Oligoclonal band negative MS
- Purely cognitive or psychiatric presentations
- Hemiplegic presentation

NB: none of these features exclude a diagnosis of MS.

Diagnostic schemes for clinical diagnosis and classification of MS   several clinically based diagnostic classifications of MS are in use, or have been used in the past[189-192] [see *Tables 7–10*]. Until recently, the most widely recognized diagnostic classification was known colloquially as the 'Poser' or 'Washington Committee' Criteria,[191] which were designed for research purposes. The most recent review by committee aimed to create criteria that could be used by the practising physician as well as by clinical trialists.[192]

Diazepam   established muscle relaxant that has been shown to reduce spasticity in MS.[115,116] Because of its sedative and habituating effects baclofen or tizanidine are preferred antispastic medications.

Diet   a possible association between animal fat intake and risk of MS has been reported.[292,293] Low MS incidence has been correlated with a high intake of vegetables, fruit and fish.[293] [See also *Polyunsaturated fatty acid diet* and *Table 12*.]

Differential diagnosis   many conditions can mimic some or all of the clinical features of MS [see *Table 13*]. In practice problems arise mainly with unusual or atypical presentations, monophasic episodes (particularly involving brainstem or spinal cord), progressive syndromes and patients presenting with an isolated lesion, cognitive deterioration, psychiatric illness or organic personality change.

Table 12 Empirical dietary treatment in MS

Diet	Rationale	Risk/costs	Conclusion
Allergen-free	The lesion of MS may be an allergic reaction to common allergens	No risk; inexpensive	No scientific basis, ineffective
Kousmine	MS occurs as a result of an unhealthy diet	Negligible	Ineffective
Gluten-free	Rates of MS relate to consumption of wheat and rye	Inadequate protein intake	Ineffective
Raw food, Evers	Illness due to unnatural methods of production and processing of foods	No risk; inexpensive	No scientific basis, ineffective
MacDougal	A combination diet was thought to be responsible for the disappearance of MacDougal's symptoms	Negligible	No scientific basis, ineffective
Pectin- and fructose-restricted	Pectin and fructose enhance autoimmunization and tissue damage	Inexpensive	No scientific basis
'Cambridge' and other liquid	No rationale for use in MS except for reduction of obesity	Significant risks	No scientific basis, not recommended
Sucrose- and tobacco-free	MS is caused by a form of allergy to sucrose or tobacco	Inexpensive	No scientific basis, unproven
Vitamins	MS may result from an unidentified vitamin deficiency	Vitamins A and D in high doses are toxic	No scientific proof, ineffective
Megavitamin therapy	MS may result from an unidentified vitamin deficiency	High doses of vitamin A, D, E and K are toxic	No scientific basis
Megascorbic therapy	MS is caused by a deficiency of vitamin C	Stomach problems and kidney stones	Unproven, not recommended
Minerals	Use of zinc phosphates in the treatment of MS	Toxic	No evidence of effectiveness
Cerebrosides	Deficiency in fatty acids might play a role in MS	Negligible	Ineffective
Aloe vera	Antibacterial and anti-inflammatory effects	Mild diarrhoea and skin hypersensitivity	Not recommended

Constructed from Polman et al.[326]

52

Table 13 Differential diagnosis of MS

Inflammatory diseases
   Systemic lupus erythematosus
   Polyarteritis nodosa
   Sjögren's disease
   Behçet's disease
   Acute disseminated encephalomyelitis
   Post infectious encephalomyelitis
   Granulomatous angiitis
   Paraneoplastic encephalomyelitis
Vascular diseases
   Prothrombotic states
   Mitochondrial encephalopathies
   CADASIL
Granulomatous diseases
   Sarcoidosis
   Wegener's granulomatosis
   Lymphomatoid granulomatosis
Infectious diseases
   Viral encephalitides
   Neuroborreliosis
   Immunodeficiency virus (AIDS)
   HTLV-I virus
   Neurosyphilis
   Progressive multifocal leukencephalopathy (PMLE)
   Whipple's disease
   Subacute sclerosing panencephalitis
Hereditary diseases
   Adrenomyeloleukodystrophy
   Metachromatic leucodystrophy
   Spinocerebellar ataxias
   Hereditary spastic paraplegia
Deficiency diseases
   Subacute degeneration of the spinal cord (B_{12} deficiency)
   Folic acid deficiency
Nonorganic (psychiatric) disease
   Hysteria
   Depression
   Somatization syndromes
   Neuroses ('fear of MS')
Other
   Congenital malformations (e.g. Arnold–Chiari, spinal dysraphism)
   Spinal tumours (e.g. meningioma or neurofibroma)
   Vascular malformations

Diffusion-weighted imaging   MRI technique based upon the microvascular water environment that is sensitive to diffusion of water molecules over short distances.[294] Pathologically damaged tissue is associated with increased diffusion of water molecules that can be detected in vivo by MRI and expressed as an increased apparent diffusion coefficient (ADC). ADC has been reported to be higher in MS plaques than in normal-looking white matter.[97,295] It is also higher in chronic plaques and lower in the peripheral rim adjacent to acute plaques, due to an increase in the extracellular space, with greater tissue destruction in the former, and cellular inflammation with oedema, in the latter. The association of brain ADC histograms with EDSS and brain atrophy suggests that diffusion imaging can provide a useful measure of total tissue integrity in MS.[296] [See also *Normal appearing white matter.*]

Diplopia   double vision or diplopia is a common symptom of brainstem lesions in MS. It may be an isolated symptom, or accompany other symptoms/signs of a brainstem lesion or long-tract involvement. It is often transient and due to involvement of the sixth nerve outflow tract, or an acute lesion in the medial longitudinal bundle (internuclear ophthalmoplegia). Less commonly it may be due to partial lesions of the third nerve outflow tract. It is reported in 29% to 39% of patients in cross-sectional studies[297] and is a presenting symptom in 8% to 22%.[62,299] Diplopia may occur as a paroxysmal symptom [see below].

Diplopia, paroxysmal   attacks of diplopia may occur in isolation or combined with paroxysmal dysarthria and ataxia. Some subjects experience symptoms up to 100 times a day, each lasting seconds to a few minutes. Paroxysmal diplopia may be explained by discharges in abducens nerve fibres within the pons, or by discharges in the medial longitudinal fasciculus.[660] [See also *Paroxysmal syndromes.*]

Disability (WHO definition)   personal limitations imposed upon the activities of daily living by neurological impairment.[300] This term has been replaced by activity limitation[5] [see also *Activity limitation*].

Disability progression   term that causes considerable confusion as it has both lay and technical meanings. Disability progression (i.e. worsening disability) in a clinical trial is usually defined by the outcome measure 'confirmed progression', which is not necessarily the same as 'progression' in real life.

Progression in real life means relentless irreversible worsening of disability, whereas 'confirmed progression', as defined in a trial, is not invariably irreversible. Irreversible worsening of disability in RR MS cohorts is difficult to ascertain over short periods of 2 to 3 years, as the median time to strong endpoints such as EDSS 6.0 takes much longer.[224,301,302] More than 5 years may be required to observe conversion to SP with confidence.[303] [See also *Confirmed progression*.]

Disability rating scales   instruments for measuring or rating the level of disability due to disease. They may be subjective, objective or mixed, generic, disease-specific or function-specific (e.g. the Ambulation Index and the Nine-Hole Peg Test are function-specific) [see *Table 14*].

Disability Status Scale (DSS)   measure designed to represent the sum of a patient's neurological dysfunction and to measure his/her maximal function

Table 14 Clinical disability rating scales

Name	Abbreviation	Reference
Disability Status Scale	DSS	304
Expanded Disability Status Scale	EDSS	305
Kurtzke Functional System Scores	KFS	306
Scripps Neurologic Rating Scale	SNRS	307
Ambulation Index	AI	29
Nine-Hole Peg Test	9HPT	146
Illness Severity Scale	ISS	308
Box and Block Test	–	146
Cambridge Basic MS Score	CAMS	151
Disease Steps	–	309
Functional Independence Measure	FIM	310
MS Functional Composite	MSFC	311
Guy's Neurological Disability Scale*	GNDS*	312
Incapacity Status Scale	ISS	313
Environmental Status Scale	ESS	313
Quantitative Neurological Examination	QNE	314
Troiano Scale	–	315

*Currently under multi-centre evaluation as the UK Neurological Disability Scale

given the neurological deficits.[304] It is an 11-point scale (0 = normal neurological examination and 10 = death due to MS) that measures overall disability. Because of insensitivity and limitations in studies of chronic MS, the Expanded Disability Status Scale (EDSS) was developed,[305] which divides each DSS step (except 0) into two.

Disconnection syndrome interruption of the connections between cerebral hemispheres through lesions in the corpus callosum, or between different parts of one hemisphere,[316] may result in a disconnection syndrome. Patients with MS, particularly those with significant callosal atrophy on MRI, may have left ear suppression on a verbal dichotic listening task and delayed naming in the left visual field on tachistoscopic object presentation.[317] Severe corpus callosum atrophy and diffuse white matter pathology may contribute to the disconnection syndrome in MS.[318] [See also *Corpus callosum.*]

Disease activity see *Gadolinium-enhancing lesion* and *T₂ active lesion.*

Disease course classification a number of attempts have been made to classify the disease course of MS according to the pattern of progression and/or relapse activity. The latest [127] recognized four different disease courses: relapsing–remitting, secondary progressive, primary progressive and progressive–relapsing. [See *Figure 12.*]

Disease duration generally measured from the first definite symptom [see also *Onset symptoms*], although in many cases the disease may have a preclinical or presymptomatic phase varying from days to many years. Needs to be carefully distinguished from disease duration from diagnosis— a period that may be very different to disease duration from first symptom (e.g. diagnosis may have been delayed for many reasons despite symptoms).

Disease onset usually defined as the date of occurrence of the first symptoms that can definitely be attributed to MS. It is considered to be a rather unreliable indicator as MRI evidence of disease may long precede symptoms, first symptoms are often forgotten, and minor or vague symptoms, not satisfying definitions of relapse, have been shown to be significant in case control studies.[320] [See also *Onset symptoms.*]

1.

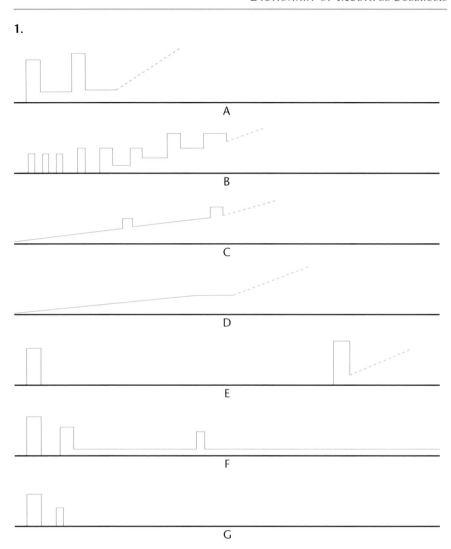

Figure 12 **Disease course classification: 1.** The Course of Multiple Sclerosis (A) Severe relapses, increasing disability and early death. (B) Many short attacks, tending to increase in duration and severity, (C) Slow progression from onset, superimposed relapses, and increasing disability, (D) Slow progression from onset without relapses, (E) Abrupt onset with good remission followed by long latent phase, (F) Relapses of diminishing frequency and severity; slight residual disability only, (G) Abrupt onset; few if any relapses after first year; no residual disability. Reproduced with permission.[644]

(*cont.*)

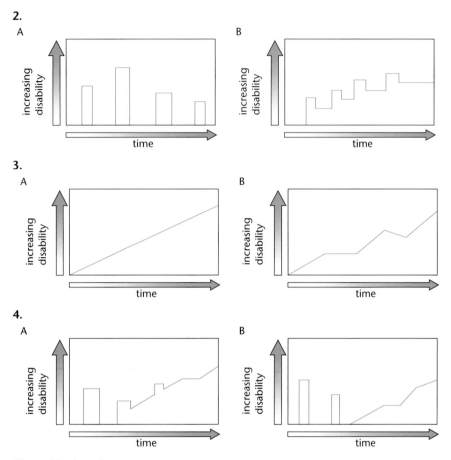

Figure 12 (*cont.*)

2. Relapsing-remitting (RR) MS is characterized by clearly defined acute attacks with full recovery* (A), or with sequelae and residual deficits (B). Note that progression of disability in RR MS thus occurs by accumulating sequelae. Periods between relapses are *usually* characterized by some improvement (as shown), and not by gradual worsening. However, a sudden stepwise deteriorating course may also occur due to relapses with little or no remission.

* New lesions and atrophy on MRI and cognitive deterioration on serial testing show that 'subclinical deterioration' (i.e. disease progression) is continuous despite lack of overt relapses.

3. Primary progressive (PP) MS is characterized by a disease course showing progression of disability from onset, without plateaus or remissions (A), or with (B) occasional plateaus and temporary minor improvements. There should be *no* evidence of a preceding phase of relapsing–remitting disease.

4. Secondary progressive (SP) MS is ushered in by the onset of a progressively deteriorating course with (A), or without (B) superimposed relapses and remissions. There must be a preceding phase of relapses and remissions as shown. Note that disability deteriorates gradually between relapses, the distinguishing feature from RR MS in which clinical deterioration is relapse-related.

(*cont.*)

5.

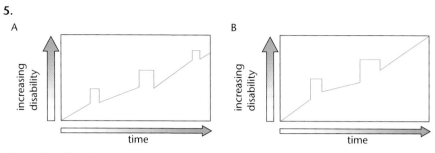

A

increasing disability

time

B

increasing disability

time

Figure 12 (*cont.*)

5. Progressive-relapsing (PR) MS shows progression from onset but with clear acute relapses with (A) or without (B) full recovery. Some of these cases may be SP MS in which evidence of a preceding phase of RR MS has been forgotten or lost.

Figs 12 (2–5) reproduced with permission.[127]

Disease Steps impairment scale focused on the assessment of ambulation. There are seven steps, including normal, mild and moderate disability, early and late use of a cane, need for bilateral support and need for a wheelchair.[309] It has a high rate of inter-rater reproducibility and is simple to administer, but is limited to ambulation assessment and is relatively subjective and imprecise.

Disseminated sclerosis old name for multiple sclerosis [see also *Multiple sclerosis*].

Dissemination in space see *Multiplicity of (separate) lesions.*

Distribution of MS see *Latitude, effects on prevalence.*

Dizygotic twins twins due to fertilization of two eggs with 50% of their genes in common.

Dying-back oligodendrogliopathy ultrastructural characteristic of oligodendrocyte dystrophy in the most distal parts of the cell processes, associated with impaired expression of myelin-associated glycoprotein. It is a typical feature of brain biopsies in early MS and may reflect impairment of oligodendrocyte metabolism in MS lesions.[11,321] [See also *Oligodendrocyte.*]

Dysaesthetic extremity pain characteristically described as a constant burning sensation, mostly in the feet, or a painful tingling or throbbing 'like a toothache', worse at night, in the heat and on walking, is the most common chronic pain syndrome encountered by MS patients.[323] It may become generalized and is often intractable. It is probably due to deafferentation of spinal cord nociceptive pathways in the dorsal columns.[323] Gabapentin has been reported to be an effective treatment.[324]

Dysarthria slurred speech due to brainstem, cerebellar, or bilateral pyramidal tract pathology, is a common symptom or sign in MS. There may be slow lateral tongue movements, associated brainstem signs or a pseudobulbar palsy with emotional incontinence and exaggerated jaw jerk. Dysarthria, often accompanied by ataxia, may also occur as a paroxysmal symptom of MS [see also *Dysarthria, paroxysmal*].

Dysarthria, paroxysmal episodes of slurred speech lasting 15–20 seconds. Attacks may be spontaneous or precipitated by movement, talking or hyperventilation.[662] There may be concurrent transient diplopia or tonic seizure.[662,663] Harrison and McGill[664] suggest that attacks of paroxysmal dysarthria and ataxia are caused by a 'build-up' of postsynaptic facilitation from an epileptic discharge around a brainstem plaque. Successful treatment with carbamazepine has been reported.[662] [See also *Paroxysmal syndromes*.]

Dyschromatopsia (achromatopsia) acquired colour vision defect of red/green perception. It is generally the first visual function to be involved in ON and the last to be restored. Small visual field defects detectable with red test objects may persist after ON ('desaturation scotoma'). The Farnsworth–Munsell '100 hue test' is superior to Ishihara plates for detecting colour vision dysfunction in optic nerve disease.[322]

Dyssynergia see *Detrusor–sphincter dyssynergia*.

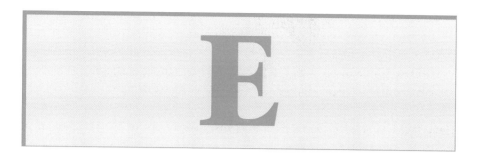

Echo time (TE)   time between the centre of the 90° pulse and the centre of the spin-echo production in MRI.

EDMUS-GS   see *European Database for MS Grading Scale.*

Effect size   standardized estimate of the magnitude of a statistically determined experimental effect, such as change over time in a group, or the difference between two groups, calculated as mean change/SD of the initial distribution of scores.[325] It is used in addition to the statistical *P* value to help interpret and compare the meaningfulness of the changes found in a study and to calculate the sample size required for a proposed study to show statistically significant changes between, or within, groups.

Empirical treatments   treatments that either have no scientific rationale, a weak rationale or a rationale that proves to be incorrect. Many suggested treatments for MS have been based on reports that a few patients had shown apparent symptomatic improvement. Some of these ineffective treatments are included in *Tables 12* (on page 52) and *15* (below).

Endothelial leukocyte adhesion molecule-1 (E-selectin)   member of the selectin family of adhesion molecules produced predominantly by activated endothelium in an inflammatory process. Its expression is induced by interleukin-1 and tumour necrosis factor-α and augmented by interferon-γ.[327] Increased CSF and serum levels of soluble E-selectin are found in MS with higher concentrations in primary progressive than relapsing–remitting or secondary progressive MS.[328,329]

Endpoint   measure of status (e.g. neurological) in the course of disease that can be used to assess the outcome or prognosis in studies of the natural history or the efficacy of a putative therapy in a trial. Different endpoints

Table 15 Some empirical treatments for MS

Treatment	Rationale	Risk/costs	Conclusion
Intravenous yeasts (Proper-Myl)	Augments body defences against infections	Mild fever	Ineffective
Pancreatic extract (Depropanex)	Vasodilator and influence on carbohydrate	Severe, sometimes life-threatening reactions	Ineffective
Snake venom (Proven, Venogen)	Contains nerve growth factor; prevents the action of a persistent virus	Pain and swelling at the injection site; severe allergic reaction	No scientific basis
Honey bee venom	Stimulates the immune system	Severe allergic reaction	No benefit
Octacosanol	Accelerates repair of damaged myelin	Negligible	No evidence of value
Superoxide dismutase (Orgotein, Orgosein, Palosein)	Attenuates experimental inflammatory demyelination	Not toxic	No evidence of effectiveness
Dimethyl sulphoxide	Immunosuppressive properties	Causes cataracts, rashes, nausea, vomiting, chills, drowsiness	No evidence of effectiveness
Alphasal (formerly cholorazone or vitamin X)	Obscure	Not known	No scientific basis
Cellular therapy	No scientific rationale	Autoimmunization and maybe death	Ineffective and dangerous
Allergens	Densensitization	Negligible; costly	Ineffective
Rodilemid	Inhibits viral infection	Low toxicity	No scientific basis
Autogenous vaccine	Vaccination	Dangerous; costs are undetermined	Not recommended
Proneut	Provocation therapy	High cost	Ineffective
Alpha-fetoprotein	Reduced relapse rates during pregnancy	Not known	No scientific basis
Immunobiological revitalization	Stimulates immune function	Not known; expensive	No scientific basis

	Therapeutic action		
Proteolytic enzymes	Therapeutic action on inflammation	Not toxic; high cost	No scientific basis
Ethylenediamine tetraacetic acid	Chelation therapy	Potentially lethal; very high cost	No scientific basis
Sodium bicarbonate, phosphates	Improves nerve conduction	Not compatible with good health	No scientific basis
Oral calcium + magnesium + vitamin D	Deficiency produces instability of myelin	Inexpensive	No scientific basis
St John's wort	Effect on brain neurochemicals	Uncertain; inexpensive	May be helpful in mild depression
Hyperimmune colostrum (immune milk)	Immunity against infections	Skin rash, mild allergic reaction	No scientific basis
Acupuncture	Relieves pain and muscle spasm	May carry the risk of hepatitis, faint, lung puncture	No scientific basis
Dorsal column stimulation	Controls pain	Infection, haemorrhage and serious spinal cord injury	Ineffective and dangerous
Hyperbaric oxygen	Improves mental function, suppresses EAE	Blindness or convulsive episodes; high cost	Ineffective
Transcutaneous nerve stimulation	Improves CNS performance	Skin irritation and dysaesthesias	No scientific basis
Thalamotomy, thalamic stimulation	Reduces tremor or other involuntary movements	Complications of brain operation; high cost	Not recommended
Sympathectomy and ganglionectomy	Increases blood supply to the CNS	Associated with major surgery; high cost	No scientific basis
Surgical spinal cord relaxation (cervicolordodesis)	Reduces abnormal pressure on nerve fibres	High risk and cost	No scientific basis
Magnetotherapy	Improves circulation, oxygenation and reduces inflammation and scarring	Not known; expensive	No scientific basis
Implantation of brain substances	No clear rationale	Dangerous and expensive	Ineffective
Hysterectomy	Progesterone induces autoimmunization	Risk of major surgery; high cost	Not recommended

have varying sensitivities and predictive reliabilities. For an endpoint to be useful as an outcome measure in a clinical trial it must be clinically relevant, sensitive and not prone to fluctuations or 'noise'.[224] It should not be erroneous through reversibility. Many endpoints have been used in MS treatment trials, including EDSS and relapse rate [see also *Outcome measure* and *Table 16*].

Enhancing lesion   see *Gadolinium-enhancing lesion*.

Enlarging T₂ lesions   lesions showing an identifiable increase in size from a previously stable-appearing lesion on a T2-weighted image.[334]

Environmental Status Scale (ESS)   handicap scale that rates personal, social, economic, employment and community functions relative to the patient's cultural norm.[313] It is comprised of 7 items: work status, financial/economic status, personal residence/home, personal assistance required, transportation, community services and social activity. Each item on the scale is scored from 0 to 5, where 0 is normal, with incremental increases in the score relative to the social and environmental impact of MS.

Environment, effects of   MS may be a place-related, acquired disease. Several lines of evidence support the environmental theory. The prevalence of MS generally increases with distance from the Equator.[335] Migration may alter the risk of occurrence of MS and the effect on risk depends on age at migration.[336,337] Offspring of immigrants often have prevalence rates similar to those in their new residence and different from their place of origin.[338] Clusters and epidemics of MS have been described,[339,340] although clustering is generally considered to be due to statistical chance.

Ependymitis, granular   see *Granular ependymitis*.

Epidemic   excess of cases over normally expected rates derived from a common or propagated source.[341] Claims have been made for MS clusters in the Faroe Islands,[342,343] Iceland,[344] Orkney and Shetland[345] and Key West.[346] Conclusions are controversial and the increased prevalence reported has been attributed to improved case ascertainment.[201,347]

Epidemic, type 1   excess cases in susceptible populations exposed for the first time to a virulent infectious agent.[348] If the entire population is exposed, the

Table 16 Endpoint measures in major phase III randomized controlled trials of immunomodulatory therapy in RR MS

Trials	IFNβ-1b[330]	IFNβ-1a (intramuscular)[331]	Glatiramer acetate[332]	IFNβ-1a (subcutaneous)[333]
Primary endpoints	1. Annual relapse rate 2. Proportion of relapse-free patients	1. Time to confirmed (6 m) worsening by 1.0 EDSS point and proportion of patients progressing	1. Mean number of relapses	1. Mean number of relapses
Secondary endpoints	1. Time to 1st relapse 2. Relapse severity 3. Relapse duration[b] 4. Mean EDSS change 5. Mean SNRS change 6. MRI outcome	1. Mean EDSS change[a] 2. Number of relapses per patient[a] 3. Upper limb function[b] 4. Lower limb function[b] 5. MS functional disability[b] 6. Comprehensive neuro-psychology battery[b] 7. CSF analysis[b] 8. MRI outcome	1. Proportion of relapse-free patients 2. Time to 1st relapse 3. Proportion of confirmed (3 m) worsening by 1.0 EDSS 4. Mean EDSS change 5. Mean AI change	1. Time to 1st and 2nd relapses 2. Proportion of relapse-free patients 3. Proportion of confirmed (3 m) worsening by 1.0 EDSS point 4. Mean AI change 5. Mean arm function score change 6. Steroid use 7. Hospital admission 8. AUC EDSS change 9. MRI outcome 10. Subgroup analysis with entry EDSS > 3.5

[a]Results reported only in the subgroup of subjects completing ≥2 years of study. m = months)
[b]Results not reported in the initial publication.

ages of those affected clinically will define the age range of susceptibility to the infection.[343,823] Post hoc cluster analysis is used for type 1 epidemic study [see also *Post hoc cluster analysis*].

Epidemic, type 2   excess cases in a population in which a virulent organism is already established.[348] A low 'age-at-onset' is characteristic as the effective exposure begins at the age of susceptibility. Space–time cluster analysis is used for type 2 epidemic studies [see also *Space–time cluster analysis*].

Episode   see *Relapse*.

Epitope   see *Antigenic determinant*.

Epitope (determinant) spreading   generation of new reactivities to new determinants on the same antigen (intramolecular) or on different antigens (intermolecular) during a prolonged immune response. Shown to be important for the pathogenesis of relapsing EAE and thought to operate in MS.[349]

E-selectin   see *Endothelial leukocyte adhesion molecule-1*.

Ethnicity   see *Race*.

ETOMS (Rebif®, Serono International SA)   the Early Treatment of MS (ETOMS) study investigated the effect of weekly subcutaneous injection of 22 μg INFβ-1a for 2 years on 308 patients who had experienced a first demyelinating event with high risk of conversion to clinically definite MS.[350] The probability of the development of clinically definite MS during a two-year follow-up period was significantly lower in the INFβ-1a treated group than in the placebo group. The relapse rates were significantly lower in the treated patients and, on MRI, both lesion activity and the accumulating lesion burden were reduced compared with placebo. [See also *OWIMS* and *PRISMS*.]

Euphoria   abnormal emotional state of elation that occurs in some MS patients, and more commonly found in association with advanced disease, high MRI lesion loads and/or dementia.[351,352]

European database for MS grading scale (EDMUS-G9)   11-point scale derived from the DSS with a short and unambiguous formulation.[353] Grade 0 describes normal status, 1 and 2 minimal signs or nonambulation related disability, 3–9 increasing ambulation related disability and 10, death due to MS. It has been formulated for clinical and epidemiological studies.

Event-related potential (ERP)   small phasic potentials elicited in conjunction with sensory, cognitive and motor events that can be de-detected by recording from scalp electrodes. ERPs are the 'far-field' reflections of patterned neural activities associated with informational transactions in the brain.[703] A high incidence of abnormal ERP has been demonstrated in MS patients.[354] Approximately 30% of patients with clinically isolated myelopathy suspected to be due to early MS may have abnormalities of memory-specific ERPs.[355] Increased P300 latency is particularly associated with poorer performance on neuropsychological testing.[356]

EVIDENCE Study (Rebif®, Serono International SA)   a comparative trial in 677 patients with RR MS in which outcomes of treatment with either once-weekly IFNβ-1a (Avonex®) or thrice-weekly IFNβ-1a (Rebif®) were compared for evidence of dose–response. All relapse and MRI outcomes were statistically in favour of the higher dose regime (Rebif three times weekly). Compared to Avonex® over 16 months, Rebif® doubled the time to first relapse $(P < 0.002)$, reduced the relapse rate by 17% $(P = 0.03)$, reduced steroid use by 32% $(P = 0.009)$, reduced T_2-lesion activity by 36% $(P < 0.001)$, reduced active scans by 38% $(P < 0.001)$ and the proportion of patients with no MRI activity by 53% $(P < 0.001)$. This study formally confirmed the dose–reponse effects of IFNβ that have been identified in most previous multidose treatment trials.[839]

Evoked potential amplitude   voltage of a waveform or peak in microvolts that is measured either from a predetermined baseline, or peak-to-peak from the preceding wave of opposite polarity. More variable than latency for clinical purposes, but within subject interocular comparisons it shows less variance and can be useful. Interocular amplitudes are commonly reduced by demyelinating lesions due to temporal dispersion, conduction block and axonal loss.

Evoked potential latency   time interval (in milliseconds) between stimulus onset and a specified point on an EP waveform (usually a peak). EP peak latencies are highly dependent on stimulus characteristics. For example, VEP latency (and amplitude) are partially dependent on luminance, contrast, colour, check size and stimulus field size. 'Delays' (or latency prolongations) are established by comparison with normal control data and are usually defined as exceeding 2.5 or 3.0 SD of the control population mean. Delayed EPs are common in MS populations, but do not necessarily imply slowed signal conduction time. EPs are compound responses and the pathological waveform is altered by partial and irregular demyelination, conduction block and axonal loss with concomitant amplitude reductions, waveform dispersion and redistribution of activity across the scalp. 'Latency comparisons' are often erroneously made between nonanalogous waves. Many apparent delays are caused by waveform alterations due to visual field defects that can be quite subtle. Other factors that can affect latency include gender, eye dominance, visual acuity, presence of ptosis, body temperature (Uhtoff's phenomenon) and variable fixation. Abnormal EP delays are nonspecific for demyelination and type of pathology.

Evoked potentials (EPs)   electrical potentials evoked by, and time-locked to, brief and abrupt sensory stimuli through specific sensory pathways (e.g. visual evoked potentials, VEPs; brainstem auditory evoked potentials, BAEPs; and somatosensory evoked potentials, SEPs). Axonal volleys generating EPs are conducted along peripheral and CNS pathways associated with the stimulated sensory modalities. EPs may be delayed, attenuated, dispersed or blocked by areas of demyelination and axonal loss.[148,357] EPs can detect 'clinically silent' lesions in specific afferent pathways and thus are useful in confirming the diagnosis of MS.[148] Many studies have demonstrated a good correlation between symptoms and signs of involvement of a given nervous pathway and the relevant EP abnormalities.[148,358,359] For all EP modalities, the frequency of abnormalities decreases with the diagnostic certainty, i.e. from definite MS to probable or possible MS cases (*Table 17*). It is rare to find normal VEPs after symptomatic optic neuritis (<5% in acute phases), but more common (20–30% normal) with sensory (SEP) and motor (MEP) pathway involvement[174,360] and with evidence of brainstem (BAEP) (50–60% normal) lesions.[361] A role for EPs has been proposed for monitoring in therapeutic trials, because they may be sensitive to progression or stability of MS over one or several years.[362–364]

Exacerbation   see *Relapse*.

Expanded Disability Status Scale (EDSS)   modified version of DSS used for rating impairment and disability in MS. It is a 20-step ordinal scale which that ranges between 0 (normal status) and 10 (death due to MS).[305] It is

Table 17 Frequency of abnormality (%) of paraclinical tests in MS (*n* = 235) according to diagnostic certainty

	VEPs	mSEPs	tSEPs	BAEPs	bMRI	CSFob
Definite	83	71	77	50	96	78
Probable	53	62	73	59	82	58
Possible	58	15	20	8	51	40
Total	73	56	62	41	83	65

VEPs = visual evoked potentials; mSEPs = median nerve somatosensory evoked potentials; tSEPs = tibial nerve somatosensory evoked potentials; BAEPs = brainstem auditory evoked potentials; bMRI = brain magnetic resonance imaging; CSFob = cerebrospinal fluid oligoclonal bands. Adapted with permission.[148]

graded according to the findings of a standard neurological examination in the appropriate grades of the functional system. It has been widely used in clinical trials of MS as a measure of disease progression,[331,333,365] despite its many imperfections. These include lack of precision,[366,367] low reliability,[368,369] uneven distribution[366,370] and low responsiveness.[312,367] It is not a pure disability scale as it measures mainly impairment in the range ≤3.5 [see *Appendix 1*].

Experimental allergic (autoimmune) encephalomyelitis (EAE) experimental animal model of demyelinating disease which was first described in 1933.[371] Active EAE arises from the immunization of experimental animals with myelin-rich tissue purified myelin proteins (including myelin basic protein, myelin oligodendrocyte glycoprotein, proteolipid protein, etc), or encephalitogenic fragments of these proteins. Passive EAE arises from adaptive transfer of activated myelin–protein reactive T cells from immunized animals to naïve animals. It is characterized by inflammatory infiltrates and demyelination in the brain and spinal cord.[372,373] Different forms may mimic chronic progressive or relapsing–remitting MS sometimes with large plaque-like lesions.[374]

Exploratory treatment trial   see *Phase II treatment trial.*

Extensor spasms   muscle spasms that characteristically cause the lower limbs to suddenly extend ('my legs kick out'). They are due to spinal cord lesions and are often more troublesome in the earlier phases of spasticity. They are seldom painful.

F

Familial aggregation any trait more common in relatives of an affected individual than in the general population due to genetic and/or environmental causes. The risk of MS in the siblings of affected individuals is 3–5% greater than the general population prevalence of 0.1%.[375,376] Increased risks range from 21–31% for monozygotic twins, 3–5% for dizygotic twins[220,377] and 3–4% for biological first-degree relatives.[378] The age-adjusted risk for full siblings is significantly higher than that for half-siblings (3.46% vs 1.32%).[379]

Farmer Quality of Life Index QoL tool for MS[380] with four sub-scales: (i) functional and economic, (ii) social and recreational, (iii) affect and 'life in general', and (iv) medical problems [see *Appendix 7*].

Fast or turbo spin echo imaging (FSE or TSE) MRI sequence that uses a 90° flip angle followed by several 180° rephasing pulses to produce several spin echoes in a given repetition time. With FSE imaging, multiple-phase encodings of the multiple echoes are performed in each repetition time. An important advantage of FSE in MS is its ability to produce thinner sections with high signal-to-noise and contrast-to-noise ratios in acquisition times similar to those required for thicker section conventional spin-echo images. The sensitivity of FSE for the detection of brain lesions in MS is probably similar to, and may be higher (because of the thinner slices) than, conventional spin-echo.[249,381,382] [See also *Fluid-attenuated inversion-recovery imaging.*]

Fatigue loss of energy is a common and disabling symptom in MS, affecting up to 87% of patients;[383] 40% of patients describe it as their worst symptom.[384] Fatigue does not correlate with levels of neurological disability or MRI abnormalities,[383,385-387] but is associated with depression.[387,388] Underlying mechanisms remain unknown, but psychosocial factors may play an important role.[385]

Fatigue Assessment Instrument   a 29-item scale that assesses quantitative and qualitative components of fatigue in general medical conditions.[389]

Fatigue Impact Scale   scale designed to assess the perceived influence of fatigue on cognitive, physical and social dimensions in patients with MS.[390]

Fatigue rating scales   scales used to determine the specific components of fatigue and their severity [see *Fatigue Impact Scale, Fatigue Severity Scale* and *Visual Linear Scale*].

Fatigue Severity Scale   series of nine graded questions aimed at addressing specific components of fatigue, including their severity and functional effect. The Fatigue Severity Scale is reported to be reliable, stable and sensitive to clinical change.[391]

Fat-suppressed spin-echo sequence   MRI sequence used to suppress fat signals and detect the small intrinsic lesions of optic nerve.[392] [See also *Frequency-selective fat-saturation sequences* and *Short inversion-time inversion-recovery sequence*.]

Fazekas diagnostic criteria, MRI   see *MRI diagnostic criteria (of Fazekas)*.

Flexor spasms   muscle spasms that characteristically flex the lower limbs. They tend to occur in more advanced cases of MS with signs of myelopathy and marked spasticity. Spasms may be triggered by sensory stimuli and are often worse at night. Associated pain may be severe. By contrast, extensor spasms are seldom painful.

Fluid-attenuated inversion-recovery imaging (FLAIR)   MRI sequence that provides heavy T_2-weighting with suppression of signals from CSF.[395] Implementations of FLAIR are usually more sensitive in detecting lesions in supertentorial regions, especially cortical/subcortical and periventricular areas, but less sensitive in the posterior fossa than FSE and conventional spin echo.[248–250]

Frequency-selective fat-saturation sequence   MRI sequence with T_2-weighting that is sensitive to intrinsic demyelinating lesions in optic nerve.[392] It may be more sensitive than the short inversion-time inversion-recovery sequence in detecting abnormal signals and gadolinium enhancement in optic nerve.[396]

Friedreich's ataxia   see *Hereditary spinocerebellar ataxia*.

Functional Assessment of MS (FAMS)   a 59-item scoring system for QoL assessments in MS based on a 28-item health-related measure for cancer patients.[397] Six subscales that show good internal consistency, test–retest reliability and construct validity are derived from it: mobility, symptoms, emotional well-being, general contentment, thinking/fatigue and family/social well-being [see *Appendix 9*].

Functional Independence Measure (FIM)   scale designed as a sensitive and comprehensive measure of brain injury that has been applied to MS to assess disability levels.[310] It has 18 items, each with a 7-point scoring system based on the type and amount of assistance required to perform basic life activities. It has been supplemented by another 12-item scale, the functional assessment measure.[398] It has high consistency, sum score inter-rater reliability, responsiveness and correlation with the EDSS, the Barthel Index, CAMS, SNRS and AI.[32,398,399] It seems useful for establishing requirements for physical care.

G

Gabapentin   anticonvulsant drug effective in relieving trigeminal neuralgia and other paroxysmal symptoms of MS.[400] The analgesic effects may be related to modulation of central pain pathways.[401]

Gadolinium diethylenetriamine pentaacetic acid (Gd-DTPA)   complex or chelate of the organic ligand DTPA and the lanthanoid metal ion Gd^{3+}, used as a contrast agent to change tissue relaxation rates and increase tissue signal intensity, or contrast between two tissues. Enhancement of white matter regions with Gd-DTPA in MS is interpreted as evidence of blood–brain barrier breakdown in areas of active inflammation. The standard dose of a gadolinium chelate is 0.1 mmol/kg intravenously. Double or triple doses are used in some studies [see also *Gadolinium-enhancing lesion*].

Gadolinium enhanced T_1-weighted images   gadolinium enhanced T_1-weighted images are used to assess and quantify disease activity in MS [see also *Gadolinium-enhancing lesion*].

Gadolinium-enhancing lesion (Gd+ lesion)   areas of high signal intensity on T_1-weighted images that appear after intravenous injection of gadolinium [see *Figure 13*]. Gadolinium-enhancing lesions indicate breakdown of the blood–brain barrier and inflammation in acute MS lesions. They tend to persist for 2 to 6 weeks, leaving behind a T_2 hyperintense lesion.[4] Approximately 50–70% of relapsing–remitting MS patients have one or more Gd+ lesion on a random cranial MRI scan regardless of clinical disease activity.[402,403] The rate of occurrence of Gd+ lesions is 5 to 30 times higher than the clinical relapse rate and more frequent during relapses than periods of remission.[4] Gd+ lesions are less frequent in SP MS patients without superimposed relapses.[404] They correlate with EDSS[405] and have prognostic implications for future disability,[406] subsequent exacerbation rate,[407,408] T_2 hyperintense lesion burden[407,408] and brain atrophy.[87–89] The number or

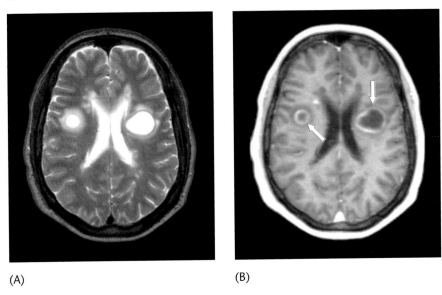

(A)   (B)

Figure 13 **Gadolinium-enhancing lesion:** A: T_2-weighted image showing lesions in clinically definite multiple sclerosis. B: T_1-weighted image from the same patient following injection of gadolinium-DTPA. Note the edges of the lesions enhance and centres do not (arrows).

volume of Gd^+ lesions is widely used as a primary endpoint for monitoring disease activity and evaluating treatment efficacy in phase II trials and as a secondary endpoint in phase III trials.[3] Steroids, interferon, glatiramer acetate, mitoxantrone, cladribine and other anti-inflammatory agents have been shown to reduce the number of Gd^+ lesions.[213,409,410]

Gender and susceptibility   most forms of MS are more common in females than males (F : M ratio 2 : 1 and 3 : 2 in different studies),[301,734] irrespective of ethnicity. The excess of females approaches 3 : 1 in children,[735] whereas MS with onset in the fifth decade or later in life, which tends to follow a primary progressive course, is more equally distributed between males and females, or even more common in males.[736]

Gender-specific rate(s)   incidence, prevalence or mortality rate(s) that relate the number of affected individuals with MS (numerators) to the proportion of the at-risk population with the same sex (denominators). This allows for variation in sex distributions between populations.

Gene   portion of a DNA molecule that is ordinarily the code for RNA transcription and usually translates into the amino-acid sequence of a particular polypeptide chain. [See also *Candidate gene.*]

Genetic complexity   preferred term for the occurrence in complex traits of complex inheritance patterns. This encompasses several forms of heterogeneity seen in single-gene disorders and adds the concept that a specific mechanism of susceptibility can have several genetic causes, which are not all operative in the same individual. Furthermore, susceptibility to a trait may consist of the aggregate of several such mechanisms.

Genetic heterogeneity   occurrence of phenotypes that appear to be the same, but have different genetic causes. There are many examples among Mendelian traits such as hereditary elliptocytosis and tuberous sclerosis.

Genetics, influence of   MS is primarily a disease of Caucasians and certain ethnic groups. Caucasians are vulnerable to MS, whereas others are resistant.[320] MS is more common in relatives of patients than in the general population.[379] The concordance of MS is 6- to 8-fold higher in monozygotic than in dizygotic twins[378] and there is an increased relative risk in full siblings[414] and half siblings.[379] There is an association with certain human leukocyte antigen genotypes.[412,413] [See also *Environment, effects of* and *HLA class II.*]

Genotype   genetic constitution of an individual, with respect either to his/her complete complement of genes, or to the allele(s) present at a particular locus.

Geographical influence   striking variations in MS prevalence around the world have been observed, with a diminishing north–south gradient in the northern hemisphere and a south–north gradient in the southern hemisphere.[415] [See *Latitude, effects on prevalence.*] (See *Table 18.*)

Glatiramer acetate (GA, copolymer 1, copaxone)   synthetic polypeptide composed of acetate salts of four amino acids, L-alanine, L-glutamic acid, L-lysine and L-tyrosine in a molar ratio of 4.2 : 1.4 : 3.4 : 1.0 (polypeptide chains with molecular weight of 4–13 kDa). GA inhibits or modifies EAE in several species exposed to encephalitogens.[416] It may be taken orally or parenterally. The injectable form is administered subcutaneously in a dose of

75

Table 18 World distribution of multiple sclerosis: Prevalence and latitude		
Location	Latitude	Prevalence*
Iceland	65°N	99.4
Shetland Islands	61°N	129.0
Winnipeg, Canada	50°N	35.0
Seattle, WA, USA	47°N	69.0
Switzerland	47°N	52.0
Parma, Italy	44°N	11.6
Arles, France	44°N	9.0
Krk, Croatia	44°N	44.0
Olmsted County, MN, USA	44°N	122.0
Copparo, Sardinia	44°N	31.0
Asahikawa, Japan	44°N	2.5
Hobart, Tasmania	43°N	68.0
Hautes Pyrenées, France	43°N	39.6
Boston, MA, USA	42°N	41.0
Sassari, Sardinia	41°N	69.0
Alcoy, Spain	39°N	17.0
Seoul, Korea	38°N	2.0
Malta	36°N	4.0
Cape Town, South Africa	36°S	
Afrikaner		10.9
'Coloured'/Oriental		3.0
Charleston, SC, USA	33°N	14.0
Newcastle, Australia	33°S	32.5
Israel (native)	32°N	
Sephardi		9.5
Ashkenazi		35.6
New Orleans, LA, USA	30°N	6.0
Kuwait (Arabs)	30°N	
Kuwaiti		9.5
Palestinian		24.0
Canary Islands	29°N	18.3
Okinawa, Japan	26°N	1.9
Hong Kong	23°N	0.8
Bombay (Parsi)	19°N	26.0

*per 100 000 inhabitants. Reproduced with permission.[844]

20 mg daily. In the US phase III study, although relapse rate was marginally reduced by active treatment (29%, $p = 0.055$), there was only a non-significant trend towards improvement of disability progression (24.8% on active treatment *vs* 15.2% on placebo, improved by ≥ 1 EDSS point).[332] During an extension of the study to 35 months, the time to progression of either ≥ 1.0 or ≥ 1.5 EDSS points (in the absence of a recent exacerbation-associated deterioration) favoured GA. The proportion of patients who worsened by ≥ 1.5 EDSS point by the end of the trial was reduced by 50% in the actively treated group,[417] but a 6-year extension study which suggested that effectiveness was sustained[418] did not include the outcome of a significant proportion of dropouts. In MRI studies, the number of accumulated Gd-enhancing and new T_2-lesions was reduced by 35%[419] and the rate of brain atrophy reduced threefold in GA-treated patients compared with placebo.[420] For mechanism(s) of action, see detailed review.[421] Side-effects include local mild skin reactions and an occasional benign systemic reaction characterized by breathlessness, tightness in the chest and palpitations. A phase III trial (CORAL) investigating the efficacy and safety of oral GA in two doses (5 mg and 20 mg daily) in active RR MS was negative and a phase III trial (PROMISE) investigating the efficacy and safety of GA in approximately 900 patients with PP MS was terminated prematurely after two years because an interim analysis failed to demonstrate any clinical efficacy.

Gliosis   repair process that follows CNS injury and is a prominent pathological feature of chronic demyelinated plaques in which reactive astrocytes constitute the major cell.[180] Gliosis in chronic lesions is associated with extensive reduction of myelin, oligodendrocytes and axons and a marked increase in extracellular space.[422] The latter may be a significant contributing factor to atrophy.[83] Glial scars, which are prominent features of MS, mainly consist of hypertrophied astrocytes.[423] [See *Figure 14*.]

Glucocorticosteroids   see *Corticosteroids or glucocorticosteroids*.

Glutethimide   piperidinedione derivative with sedative–hypnotic and anticholinergic effects. One uncontrolled study suggested some efficacy in treating cerebellar tremor.[424] It is not widely used.

Granular ependymitis   small, dome-shaped areas of inflammation on the ependymal surface of the ventricles, particularly in the lateral ventricles, that probably reflect the involvement of the ependyma in inflammatory, healing

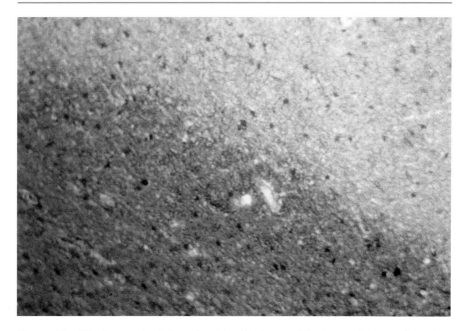

Figure 14 **Gliosis:** On the left, a chronic MS plaque with dense gliosis, and on the right macroscopically normal-appearing white matter with low-level gliosis. Immunocytochemcial staining with anti-glial fibrillary acidic protein antibody, magnification ×110. *(Courtesy of Dr J Newcombe, Institute of Neurology, London.)*

or sclerotic processes in the chronic plaques of MS.[425] The pathogenesis may be due to failure of the astrocyte-derived ependymal cells to repair after injury or to ventricular dilatation induced by sclerosis, or to shrinkage around periventricular plaques of MS.[407]

Guy's Neurological Disability Scale (GNDS) patient-reported, multidimensional scale that assesses 12 domains of MS disability, each with a point scoring system from 0 (normal) to 5 (maximum help required).[312] The categories include cognition, mood, vision, speech, swallowing, upper limb function, lower limb function, bladder function, bowel function, sexual function, fatigue and 'other'. Patients' self-reports on GNDS correlate well with neurologists' ratings on EDSS and MSFC and offer a valuable way to document disease impact in MS, but are an inadequate screen of cognitive function.[426] Further multicentre validation studies are in progress and the scale will be renamed the United Kingdom Neurological Disability Scale (UKNDS) [see *Appendix* 5].

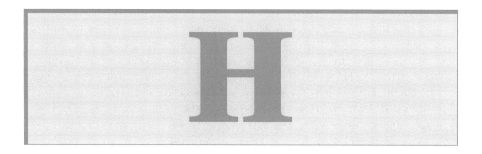

Handicap social and environmental effects of disability.[300] This term has been replaced by the term participation [see also *Participation (WHO definition)*].

Haplotype set of alleles at a group of linked genes together in a specific chromosomal region.

Health-Related Quality of Life (HRQL) tool to assess how a health problem and its treatment affect an individual's ability to perform activities and roles that she/he values.[427] It can be divided into generic and disease-specific measures. Generic measures include Sickness Impact Profile,[428] Nottingham Health Profile,[429] and the Short Form Health Survey (SF-36) from the Medical Outcomes Study.[430] The MS-specific Minimal Record of Disability is used to supplement the generic measures in HRQL [see also *Minimal Record of Disability*].

Hereditary spinocerebellar ataxia (Friedreich's ataxia) degenerative disease characterized by various combinations of gait ataxia, dysarthria, sensory and cerebellar incoordination, sensory loss, pyramidal signs and areflexia, often with a positive family history. The onset is gradual and at variable age. Pes cavus, absent ankle jerks and scoliosis are often present.[431]

HLA see *Human leukocyte antigen*.

HLA class I protein receptor expressed on the surface of almost all cells and responsible for presenting antigen to HLA class I-restricted T cells that express CD8+. [See also *CD8+ T cells*.]

HLA class II protein encoded by three sets of genes in the HLA-D region and restrictively expressed, mainly on monocytes, macrophages and B lymphocytes. These proteins are involved in communications between cells that are necessary to execute the immune response. In particular, they are required for CD4+ helper T cell function. HLA class II molecules contain HLA-DR, DQ and DP subregions. Population studies have shown that the HLA class II phenotypes DR15 and DQ6 and their corresponding genotypes DRB1*1501, DRB5*0101 and DQA1*0102, DQB2*0602 confer susceptibility to MS.[70,413,432,433] Associations have been identified with respect to other geographical, ethnic populations.[434] [See also *Association analysis*, *CD4+ T cells* and *Trimolecular complex*.]

Hot bath test   test for central demyelination in which central body temperature is raised in a bath of hot water in order to detect transient temperature-sensitive focal neurological symptoms or signs.[435] Temperature-related symptoms or signs are attributed to a heat-linked blockade (conduction block) in partially demyelinated axons.[436] The heat-induced deficits typically resolve with return of body temperature to normal, although rarely, persistent dysfunction may ensue.[437]

HTLV-I associated myelopathy   disease predominantly of the spinal cord caused by human T-lymphotropic virus type I (HTLV-I). May closely mimic chronic progressive MS.[438] Pain in the back and legs is common at onset with early bladder symptoms. Spastic weakness and sensory abnormalities are found in the lower limbs. Examination of serum for HTLV-I antibodies is crucial for diagnosis. Periventricular and deep white-matter lesions are frequently encountered in HTLV-I, but infratentorial lesions are distinctly uncommon.[291]

Hu23F2G   see *Anti-CD11/CD18 antibodies*.

Human leukocyte antigen (HLA)   cluster of genes located on the short arm of chromosome 6 that encodes several families of proteins including the class I (HLA-A, HLA-B and HLA-C) and class II molecules (HLA-DR, HLA-DQ and HLA-DP). These proteins are cell-surface glycoproteins with a central role in the regulation of the immune response. It is the first, and perhaps the only candidate region shown to encode alleles that confer susceptibility to MS.[439] [See *Candidate gene* and *HLA class II*.]

Humoral immune response   major component of the immune system characterized by the production of antibodies specific for antigenic determinants on foreign pathogens[173] or self-antigens in autoimmune conditions [see also

Autoantibody]. Although MS is associated with a T-cell-mediated inflammatory response, antibodies may play a role in pathogenesis.[440–442] Autoantibodies to several myelin proteins including MBP,[443] PLP,[443,444] MAG[445] and MOG[441] may be present in MS, but their role in disease pathogenesis is unclear. Antibodies may even play a protective role (rationale for the use of normal human immunoglobulins in MS).

Hypointense T$_1$-lesions   see *Black holes*.

Hyperintense T$_2$-lesions   see *Total lesion load*.

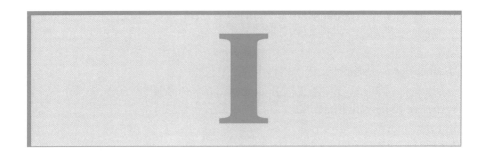

IgG index parameter recommended for the demonstration of an IgG elevation in CSF due to synthesis within the CNS, eliminating the variations in serum IgG and individual variation related to bood–brain barrier dysfunction[194]. The IgG index is the CSF/serum IgG quotient divided by the CSF/serum albumin quotient. A value of more than 0.73 is abnormal and present in 92% of patients with CD MS.[446] [See also *Oligoclonal bands.*]

Illness Severity Scale sum of weights corresponding to ratings of the Kurtzke Disability Status Scale and Functional System Scores and phase of illness (relapsing, remitting and progressive, or progressive).[308] Although criticized as complicated, unwieldy and unsuitable,[366] it has been used in one therapeutic trial.[108]

Immediate memory see *Short-term memory* and *Working memory.*

Immunogen see *Antigen.*

Immunoglobulin (Ig) mature B lymphocyte product synthesized in response to stimulation by an antigen. There are five classes of immunoglobulins (IgG, IgM, IgA, IgD and IgE). Each Ig unit is made up of two heavy and two light chains and has two antigen binding sites. IgG has four subclasses (IgG_{1-4}). IgM and IgG (in particular IgG_3) bind and activate complement. [See also *Intravenous immunoglobulin* and *Oligoclonal bands.*]

Immunoglobulin gene gene family encoded on chromosome 14 that is highly polymorphic with variable (V), diversity (D), joining (J) and constant (C) segments. Association between MS susceptibility and GM locus, a highly polymorphic region of the heavy chain of IgG, has been reported in some,[450,451] but not all studies.[452,453]

Impairment (WHO definition)   loss or abnormality of body structure or of a physiological or psychological function.[5]

Impotence   see *Sexual dysfunction.*

Imuran   see *Azathioprine.*

Incapacity Status Scale (ISS)   scale designed to grade disability. A total score is calculated on the ratings of 16 functions, including ambulation, activities of daily living, vision, speech and hearing, neuropsychological function, sphincter and sexual function, and fatigue.[313] Each item is graded on a 5-point scale where 0 = normal and 4 = loss of function. The scale is not sensitive enough to detect minor changes in clinical status.

Incidence rate   number of patients with disease onset per 100 000 population at-risk during a specified time period.[320] Subjects of different ethnic background, or with symptoms of MS when they moved to the study area, are excluded.[201]

Integrin   important mediator of immune cell migration into the CNS in inflammatory diseases.[454] The binding of integrin and its receptor VCAM-1 on the vascular endothelium facilitates leukocyte trafficking to the site of inflammation. Antibodies against α-4 integrin are effective in EAE models[455] and MS.[39] [See also *Anti-α4 integrin antibody.*]

Intention-to-treat analysis   method of analysis that includes results from patients who discontinue treatment for any reason (e.g. adverse events). These patients are followed up as if they continued on treatment and their data are then included in the statistical analysis in order to reduce bias and provide a more realistic picture of efficacy in a real-life clinical setting. Although generally considered a conservative analysis, this is not invariably the case.

Intercellular adhesion molecule-1 (ICAM-1)   member of the immunoglobulin supergene family expressed on various cells, including peripheral blood lymphocytes, endothelial cells and thymic cells. ICAM-1 is involved in adhesion of neutrophils, lymphocytes and other cells bearing the lymphocyte-function-associated antigen receptor.[19] It is markedly upregulated by cytokines generated in the course of an inflammatory process and shed from activated endothelial cells and lymphocytes.[18] Elevated levels of soluble ICAM-1 in both the serum and the CSF of patients with MS may correlate with disease activity,[20,456–458] suggesting that soluble ICAM-1 may be a marker of acute inflammation.

Interferon (IFN)   family of cytokines that interfere with viral replication. Two types of IFNs have been identified by their functional and molecular characteristics: type I (IFN-α and IFN-β) and type II (IFN-γ). IFN-α and -β are produced by almost all mammalian cells upon stimulation.[21] Both IFN-α and -β have shown efficacy in the treatment of RR MS.[331,459,460] IFN-γ, a pro-inflammatory cytokine produced by activated T cells and natural killer cells, has been associated with MS worsening.[461] [See also *Interferon alpha, Interferon beta* and *Interferon gamma*.]

Interferon alpha (IFN-α)   anti-inflammatory cytokine with antiviral and immunomodulatory properties, synthesized by almost all mammalian cells following exposure to viral proteins or synthetic nucleotides.[462] Patients with MS show a deficit in the ability to produce IFN-α[463] and an elevation of IFN-α production has been associated with clinical remissions following relapses.[464] Administration of natural and recombinant IFN-α reduces relapse rate and decreases lymphocyte IFN-γ production.[465,466]

Interferon beta (IFN-β)   anti-inflammatory cytokine, one of the type I interferons produced by almost all stimulated mammalian cells, particularly fibroblasts, macrophages and epithelial cells. Recombinant IFN-β is an established treatment for relapsing MS. Three interferon beta products are available (*Table 19*). The multicentre, placebo-controlled trials for each product have demonstrated that IFN-β decreases the number of relapses in patients with RR MS. This reduction in disease activity is associated with a striking effect on abnormalities detected by MRI. The actions of IFN-β are multiple and complex.[467] [See also *Interferon beta-1a* and *Interferon beta-1b*.]

Interferon beta-1a (IFNβ-1a; Rebif; Avonex)   recombinant form of IFNβ produced by mass tissue culture technology using a Chinese hamster ovarian cell line. It has an identical molecular structure to natural human interferon and the same pharmacological profile in healthy volunteers.[468] Several phase II or III trials have now reported on the use of once or thrice weekly IFNβ-1a. [See *CHAMPS, ETOMS, EVIDENCE, MSCRG, OWIMS, PRISMS* and *SPECTRIMS* Trials.]

Table 19 Available IFN-β products

	Rebif®	Avonex™	ªBetaseron®
Type	IFNβ-1a	IFNβ-1a	IFNβ-1b
Cell origin	CHO	CHO	E coli
Amino acid	166	166	165[b]
Glycoprotein	Yes	Yes	No
Specific activity[c]	27×10^7	27×10^7	2×10^7
Formulation	Liquid PFS	FD	FD
Weekly dose (µg)	66–132	30	875
Route of administration	Subcutaneous	Intramuscular	Subcutaneous

[a]Known as Betaseron in North America and Betaferon in the rest of the world.
[b]Absent N-methyl, position 17 Cys → Ser.
[c]IU/mcg by bioassay.
CHO, Chinese hamster ovary cells; PFS, prefilled syringe; FD, freeze-dried.

Reproduced with permission.[467]

Interferon beta-1b (IFNβ-1b; Betaseron; Betaferon)   a genetically modified ('mutant') molecule produced by *Escherichia coli* that differs from natural IFN-β and IFNβ-1a by two amino acids and the lack of a glycosylated side chain. In the first major study in MS, IFNβ-1b significantly reduced the exacerbation rate, markedly decreased new lesion formation and lesion burden on MRI, but failed to show an effect on disability progression.[330,409] (*Table 20*). In some patients who continued in an extension, beneficial effects on relapses and MRI persisted in those on 8 MIU with a trend for less disability progression.[459] It was found that 38% of patients had developed neutralizing antibodies to the drug, and these patients seemed to have much less clinical and MRI efficacy.[469] Subsequently, a large European study suggested that IFNβ-1b could slow the time to confirmed progression in SP MS[470] and reduce the activity and lesion burden on MRI.[410] However, this trial had a larger than expected proportion of patients who were actively relapsing. By contrast, the subsequent larger North American study of IFNβ-1b in more advanced cases of SP MS showed no beneficial effect on disability progression.[471]

Interferon gamma (IFN-γ)   pro-inflammatory cytokine produced by activated Th1 cells and natural killer cells that is thought to play a key role in the CNS inflammation in MS. Serum levels may be significantly elevated[472]

Table 20 Interferon beta-1b in RR MS: 2- and 3-year data

Outcome measures	Time (years)	Placebo	1.6 MIU	8 MIU	P Value*
Number of patients	2	112	111	115	—
	3	123	125	124	—
Mean exacerbation rate	2	1.27	1.17	0.84	0.0001
	3	1.21	1.05	0.84	0.0004
Mean time to first exacerbation (days)	3	147	199	264	0.028
Mean moderate and severe exacerbation rate	2	0.45	0.32	0.23	0.002
MRI BOD (median percent change from baseline)	1	10.9	3.0	−6.2	<0.001
	2	16.5	11.4	0.8	<0.001
	3	15.0	0.2	9.3	0.002

*P values are for comparison of placebo to 8 MIU; MIU = million international unit; table adapted with permission.[842]

and augmented prior to the onset of a new relapse.[464] An increased IFN-γ mRNA expression in mononuclear cells in blood and CSF has also been reported.[473] IFN-γ has been shown to induce oligodendrocyte death by apoptosis.[474] Because of the report of deficient IFN-γ production in MS patients,[475] IFN-γ was tested in a therapeutic trial. However, this resulted in an increased exacerbation rate and premature termination of the trial.[461]

Interferon-γ-inducing factor   see *Interleukin 18.*

Interleukin 1 (IL-1)   major pro-inflammatory cytokine produced by macrophages and microglial cells in and around the edge of MS lesions.[476] It activates lymphocytes and plays a role in initiating an immune response. It has been found to be increased in the CSF of MS patients and may be involved in the destruction of CNS myelin.[476,477]

Interleukin 2 (IL-2)   pro-inflammatory cytokine associated with Th1 cells and released by activated T cells.[478] IL-2 has been reported to be elevated in MS serum[479–481] and present in MS brain lesions.[482] The levels of soluble IL-2 receptor have also been found to be elevated in MS serum[481,483–485] as well as in CSF.[485–487] Elevated levels of IL-2 and IL-2 receptor in MS have been correlated with clinical relapse rate and disease duration.[485]

Interleukin 4 (IL-4)   cytokine produced preferentially by Th2 cells that assists B cells in the production of antibody.[488] IL-4 may be undetectable in CSF and serum.[487] There are reports of elevated serum IL-4 in MS patients in the acute phase alongside Th1 cytokines,[472] but also reports of decreased Vα24 cells that produce early IL-4.[489] Elevated numbers of IL-4 mRNA-expressing MNCs have been reported in blood and CSF.[473,490] The role of IL-4 in MS is unclear, but it might reduce CNS inflammation via inhibition of IFN-γ synthesis.[491] [See also *Interferon gamma* and *T-helper-2 cells.*]

Interleukin 10 (IL-10)   anti-inflammatory cytokine secreted by lymphocytes which can inhibit the synthesis of many Th1-cell-related pro-inflammatory cytokines.[492] Decreased production of IL-10 prior to exacerbations[493] and during remissions[494] has been reported. Significantly low levels of IL-10 mRNA expression and IL-10-secreting cells have been demonstrated in both RR and SP MS patients compared with controls.[495,496] IFNβ-1a increases CSF IL-10 levels[497,498] and IL-10-secreting cells[495] in MS, suggesting that normalization of IL-10 may be a mechanism underlying the beneficial effects of this treatment.

Interleukin 12 major cytokine of cell-mediated immunity. It is a heterodimer of p40 and p35 subunits that induces Th1. Elevated in the serum and the CSF of MS patients and expressed in MS brain. Neutralization of IL-12 suppresses EAE.

Interleukin 17 pro-inflammatory cytokine made by T cells that activates fibroblasts and endothelial cells.

Interleukin 18 (interferon-γ-inducing factor) pro-inflammatory cytokine made by antigen-presenting cells that induces Th1.

Interleukin 19, 20, 21, 22 cytokines all related in part to IL-10 and presumed largely anti-inflammatory.

Interleukin 23 pro-inflammatory cytokine; heterodimer of p40 (same as IL-12 p40) and p19 subunits. Increases production of interferon-γ.

Internode length of nerve fibre covered by one Schwann cell. The length of the internode is between 0.5 and 2 mm—greater for thicker fibres.

Internuclear ophthalmoplegia (INO) disorder of eye movement due to a lesion in the medial longitudinal fasciculus (MLF) which is characterized by impaired (paretic or slowed) adduction on the side of a lesion and horizontal nystagmus in the opposite, abducting eye ('ataxic nystagmus').[499] It is the most common oculomotor manifestation of MS.[500]

Intrathecal IgG synthesis production of CSF IgG synthesized by plasma cells or B lymphocytes inside the BBB,[501] is evidence of inflammation in the CNS and a feature of MS.[502] Isoelectric focusing of contemporaneous serum and CSF samples is the usual method, but some patients may have raised IgG/albumin ratios and negative OCB.[195] [See also *Oligoclonal bands.*]

Intrathecal IgG synthesis rate IgG in mg/day in the CSF derived from extravascular sources, i.e. synthesized inside the blood–brain barrier. The formula used to calculate the daily rate of synthesis is:

$$\left[\left(IgG_{CSF} - \frac{IgG_{serum}}{369}\right) - \left(Alb_{CSF} - \frac{Alb_{serum}}{230}\right) \times \left(\frac{IgG_{serum}}{Alb_{serum}}\right)(0.43)\right] \times 5$$

where IgG_{CSF} is the IgG concentration (mg/dl) in the patient's CSF; IgG_{serum} is the patient's serum IgG concentration (mg/dl); $IgG_{serum}/369$ is the IgG that is expected to cross the normal BBB from the serum to the CSF, based on the serum IgG concentration. $Alb_{CSF} - (Alb_{serum}/230)$ represents the excess of CSF albumin that has crossed a dysfunctional BBB. This term is then multiplied by $(IgG_{serum}/Alb_{serum}) \times 0.43$ to convert the excess CSF albumin to excess CSF IgG that has crossed the damaged barrier with the albumin, assuming passive transport of one mole of IgG for one mole of albumin. To calculate the daily intrathecal IgG synthesis rate (mg/day), this entire equation is then multiplied by 5 to convert from concentration in mg/dl to mg/day, since an average of 5 dl of CSF is formed each day.

Intravenous immunoglobulin (IVIg) immunoglobulins extracted from human plasma are used as immunomodulatory agents in a variety of disorders of the nervous system. In a small phase III study of RR MS, active therapy reduced the annual rate of relapses by 59% and was associated with lower disability scores compared with placebo-treated cases.[503,504] Although IVIg treatment reduced the mean number of new and total gadolinium-enhanced lesions by approximately 60% compared with placebo in a small study,[505] no parallel MRI data from larger clinical trials in RR MS are available. IVIg treatment may reduce the risk of exacerbations in the vulnerable three- to six-month postpartum period.[506] The mechanism of action in MS remains uncertain.[507] A large multicentre placebo-controlled study of IVIg in SP MS was negative and a phase III trial of IVIg in RR MS is planned.

Isolated brainstem syndrome an acute or subacute brainstem syndrome is a common initial presentation of MS[62] with diplopia, vertigo, ataxia, nystagmus, internuclear ophthalmoplegia, sixth or seventh nerve palsy, impaired trigeminal sensation and horizontal conjugate gaze palsy,[12] either alone or in various combinations, depending on the site and extent of the lesion. The risk of developing MS with such an onset has been reported to be 57% after a mean interval of 15 months.[12] The risk is increased by other MRI abnormalities, including the presence of HLA-DR2 and the demonstration of oligoclonal bands in the CSF.[12,14]

Isoniazid drug with reported efficacy in several small studies for a minority of MS patients with action[508] or postural tremor.[509] Some studies have failed to find any effects, particularly for intention tremor. It is used in doses of 800–1200 mg/day and is associated with significant hepatotoxicity.

Isoprinosine   physicochemical complex of inosine with the para-acetami-dobenzoic acid salt of N-dimethylamino-2-propanolol. Although it enhances B lymphocyte activity, it has not been shown to be an effective therapy for MS.[510]

Itching (pruritus)   unpleasant, intense itching of one or more sensory segments, usually in the limbs, is occasionally (approximately 5% of patients) observed as a symptom of MS.[319] Sensory alterations are sometimes present in the affected area. Itching may also occur as a paroxysmal symptom. [See below.]

Itching, paroxysmal   paroxysms of itching each lasting several minutes and not relieved by scratching, may be precipitated by movement or sensory stimulation and can occur many times each day. [See also *Paroxysmal syndromes.*]

J

Juxtacortical lesion lesions situated on the boundary between the white and grey matter are common in MS and constitute about 17% of cerebral plaques.[841] These lesions appear to involve selectively the subcortical U-fibres following the corticomedullary margins and are readily identified on MRI. The presence of juxtacortical lesions in patients with monosymptomatic neurological disease may be a highly specific prognostic indicator of the risk of future progression to CD MS.[118] [See *Figure 15.*]

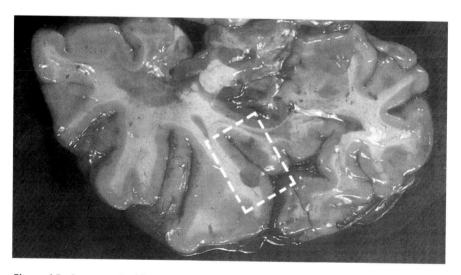

Figure 15 **Juxtacortical lesion:** Unfixed brain with MS lesions situated on the boundary between white and cortical grey matter. For full-colour version, please see accompanying CD. *(Courtesy of Dr J Newcombe, Institute of Neurology, London.)*

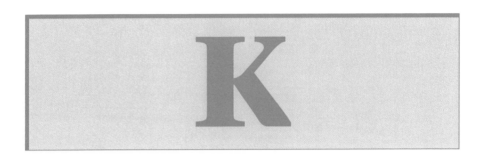

Kurtzke Functional System Scores (KFS) eight subscales that aim to measure the neurological function in eight different systems and are accumulated to provide the EDSS.[306] The functional systems are pyramidal, cerebellar, brainstem, sensory, bowel and bladder, visual, cerebral or mental, and other or miscellaneous functions. All but the last are graded from 0 (normal) to maximal impairment (grade 5 or 6). [See *Appendix 1.*]

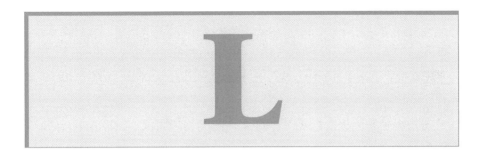

Laboratory support   term applied in the Poser criteria[191] to the finding of oligoclonal bands and/or increased production of immunoglobulin G in the CSF. Other laboratory procedures, such as evoked potentials or imaging techniques, are considered to be extensions of the clinical examination. [See *Table 9*.]

Laboratory-Supported Definite MS (LSD MS)   category in the Poser criteria[191] that requires the demonstration of IgG oligoclonal bands in CSF, or increased CNS synthesis of IgG. Oligoclonal bands must not be present in the patient's serum, and the serum IgG level must be normal. The diagnostic evidence includes:

  (i) two attacks, either clinical or paraclinical evidence of one lesion and CSF OB/IgG;
 (ii) one attack, clinical evidence of two separate lesions and CSF OB/IgG;
(iii) one attack, clinical evidence of one lesion and paraclinical evidence of another, separate lesion and CSF OB/IgG.

The two attacks must involve different parts of the CNS and be separated by a minimum of one month, each having lasted at least 24 hours. One of the episodes must involve a part of the CNS distinct from that in which abnormalities have been demonstrated from clinical or paraclinical evidence. [See *Table 9*.] Note that the newer McDonald et al[192] criteria have excluded this useful category.

Laboratory-Supported Probable MS (LSP MS)   category in the Poser diagnostic criteria[191] that requires two attacks and positive CSF OB and/or raised IgG. The two attacks must involve different parts of CNS, must be separated by a minimum of one month, and each must have lasted at least 24 hours [see *Table 9*]. Note that the term of 'probable MS' has been superseded in the latest classification.[192]

Larmor frequency frequency at which magnetic resonance can be induced in a given magnetic field. For protons (hydrogen nuclei), the Larmor frequency is 42.58 MHz/T. The corresponding variation of the Larmor frequency can be used to encode position by varying the magnetic field in one direction.

Latent MS Diagnostic category in the classification scheme of McDonald and Halliday.[190] [See *also Diagnostic criteria, clinical (McDonald and Halliday)*.]

Latitude, effects on prevalence prevalence rates have been broadly classified into low, medium and high.[692] High risk areas (>30/10^5) include northern Europe, northern USA, Canada, southern Australia, and New Zealand, medium-risk (5–30/10^5) southern Europe, southern USA and northern Australia and low risk areas (<5/10^5) Asia, Africa and South America. The direct relationship between the prevalence of MS and latitude in Europe has diminished with the finding of a higher prevalence in southern Europe (e.g. Italy) than was previously recognized.[695] Genetic factors play an important role in determining distribution in Europe and the USA (i.e. Scandinavian and northern European heritage),[695,696] but exert only a small influence on the prevalence gradient in the Southern Hemisphere (i.e. Australia and New Zealand).[697] It is clear that both genetic susceptibility and environmental influences affect the acquisition of the disease.[320,698] [See also *Genetics, influence of*.]

LD mapping localization of genes by the recognition of disease haplotypes that carry a susceptibility allele.

Leber's hereditary optic neuropathy inherited disorder transmitted through the female line. Affected males suffer from a characteristic sudden deterioration of vision, either bilaterally and simultaneously, or episodically with brief intervals, with subsequent progressive visual failure. The optic discs may be swollen and hyperaemic initially, but soon become atrophic. Central vision is affected before peripheral vision and there are bilateral scotomata. Diagnostic difficulties arise when visual symptoms are (rarely) associated with disseminated neurological signs and symptoms.[511] Mitochondrial DNA mutations, with the most common point mutation at position 11778 of mtDNA, are found to be associated with affected families.[512,513]

Lenercept (sTNFR-IgG p55) recombinant TNF receptor p55 immunoglobulin fusion protein that protects against EAE.[514,515] In one phase II clinical trial, patients treated with Lenercept experienced more exacerbations and more severe neurological deficits than patients receiving placebo.[516]

Lesion   see *Plaque*.

Lesion activity, MRI   pathologically active lesions may be defined on MRI scans by gadolinium-DTPA enhancement, which implies blood–brain barrier leakage and associated inflammation [see also *Gadolinium-enhancing lesion*]. Lesion activity is also defined as new or enlarging lesions on serial T_2-weighted imaging [see also *T_2 active lesion*].

Lesion activity, pathology   pathologically defined by, either the inflammatory reaction, or the state of myelin degradation products within macrophages in the lesion. Criteria used to define inflammatory activity are diffuse infiltration of the vessel walls and CNS parenchyma by inflammatory cells, the increased expression of histocompatibility antigens or adhesion molecules, and the definition of the activation stage of lymphocytes and macrophages in the lesions, of which myelin degradation products in macrophages is considered the best and most precise method to evaluate lesion activity.[517] [See also *Lesion activity, MRI*.]

Leukodystrophies   diseases predominantly of childhood that are unlikely to be confused with MS. Dominantly inherited adult-onset leukodystrophy with signs of spinal cord and cerebellar disease may resemble chronic progressive MS.[518] MRI typically shows diffuse rather than discrete abnormalities in white matter.

Leukotrienes (LTs)   highly potent tissue mediators and/or modulators of inflammatory processes.[519] Two types, LTB_4 and LTC_4, are recognized. Higher levels of LTB_4 and LTC_4 have been reported in the CSF of patients with MS, perhaps due to increased penetration through the blood–brain barrier and/or synthesis within the blood–brain barrier and cerebral nervous tissue.[520,521]

Levamisole   agent that regulates cell-mediated immunity by restoring T-cell function. Levamisole reduced the number of relapses during a 4-year trial,[522] but failed to do so in other studies.[523,524]

Lhermitte's sign   brief sensations, variously described as tingling, vibrating pain or electric shock-like feelings travelling down the spine, often into one

95

or both legs, and less commonly, into the arm(s), which occur suddenly on neck flexion.[525] Movement or coughing may also provoke the symptom. The sensations are often transient, resolving after a few weeks, but recurrences are frequent; 38% of patients with MS experience this symptom at some time.[526] Recent studies indicate an association with MRI abnormalities of the cervical spinal cord.[527] The sign is not specific for MS and may be secondary to a variety of different pathologies (e.g. tumours or spondylosis) that may require exclusion.

Libido   see *Sexual dysfunction.*

Lifetime risk (cumulative frequency)   maximum chance that MS will occur at any time during the life of an individual. The approximately estimated lifetime risk is $1 : 400$ for northern Europeans and $1 : 800$ for UK subjects. The risk of development of MS in a sibling of an affected patient is approximately $1 : 20$, or in an offspring, $1 : 50$. For monozygotic twins (without MRI data) the risk is $1 : 4$, or by taking presymptomatic MRI abnormalities into account, $1 : 3$.[434]

Linkage   describes the tendency of alleles at different loci to be inherited together as a result of their proximity on the same chromosome. This was first shown by Haldane for the X-linked traits haemophilia and colour blindness, using data from families. It is measured by the percentage recombination between loci and this value is given the term ' theta'. This is not necessarily the correct term for disease associations with alleles in complex traits.

Linkage analysis   technique designed to determine whether polymorphic markers cosegregate with the disease within families. Several linkage studies have shown that DR2 (DR15) within HLA class II molecule confers susceptibility to MS.[432,433,528] Although results are commonly interpreted as showing linkage, the results can be mimicked by any allele that serves to increase susceptiblity. Linkage analysis should be corrected for known allelic associations [see also *HLA class II*].

Linkage disequilibrium (LD)   tendency for an allele, disease or trait to associate with another allele more often than expected by chance. Also called allele association. The degree of LD varies tremendously throughout the genome and is very strong within the MHC. LD maps have been created indicating that LD may be strong in a region, but still contain areas that have little or no LD. [See also *LD mapping*.]

Linomide   see *Roquinimex*.

Lioresal   see *Baclofen*.

Locus   position on a chromosome at which the gene for a particular trait resides. A locus may be occupied by any one of the alleles for the gene.

Lod score   measure of genetic linkage that tests a set of linkage data and indicates whether two loci are linked or unlinked. The lod score is the base 10 logarithm of the odds-favouring linkage. A lod score of +3 (1000 : 1 odds for) is taken as proof of linkage. By consensus a score of −2 (100 : 1 odds against) is taken to indicate no linkage.

London Handicap Scale   instrument for assessing generic health status and handicap specifically designed for patients with progressive disease.[529] It is a six-item, self-report questionnaire based on the dimensions of the WHO description of handicap.[5] It is reported to have moderate to high internal consistency, good inter-rater and test–retest reliability and responsiveness. It can only be used to compare groups and should not be used to evaluate individual patients.[530]

Long-term memory (LTM)   neuronal system that makes a permanent record of an individual's experience and knowledge. Tulving[531] proposed the existence of two complementary LTM systems, episodic memory and semantic memory. Episodic memory is autobiographical in nature, consisting of memories of life events or episodes set in a spatiotemporal context (a specific time and place). Semantic memory, on the other hand, consists of knowledge of the world (e.g. facts, concepts, vocabulary), independent of the context in which the knowledge was initially learned. Performance on verbal fluency tests provides a measure of access to semantic memory. MS patients are consistently impaired on such tests.[203,204,207]

Lumbar puncture (LP, spinal tap)   insertion of a needle into the subarachnoid space, most usually via the intervertebral space between L4/L5 or L3/L4, to obtain CSF for analysis. The most common tests on the CSF are cell count, total protein estimation, glucose level and immunoglobulin determination. CSF pressure can be measured with a manometer.

Lyme disease a spirochaetal infection caused by the tick, *Borrelia burgdorferi*. Skin lesions (erythema chronicum migrans) and an acute febrile reaction following a bite by the tick usually precede a wide variety of neurological manifestations, particularly meningitis, cranial neuritis and radiculopathy. Constitutional disturbance is more marked and CSF cell count often higher than is acceptable for MS. MRI can be normal in milder forms or show bilateral periventricular white matter signal abnormalities. Antibodies to the organism are usually present.[532]

Lymphotoxin (LT-α, TNF-β) lymphokine produced predominantly by Th1 cells, but also by other cells including astrocytes.[533] It is very similar to TNF and binds the same receptor. Lymphotoxin has been demonstrated together with TNF-α in MS brain lesions.[534] The levels of LT-expressing cells are elevated in blood and CSF prior to and during MS exacerbations.[493,535] Lymphotoxin induces oligodendrocyte damage in vitro.[536] In concert with TNF-α it could contribute to demyelination in MS. There is a positive correlation between LT-α and TNF-α mRNA-expressing blood mononuclear cells in MS.[535] Like TNF-α it is not required for EAE.

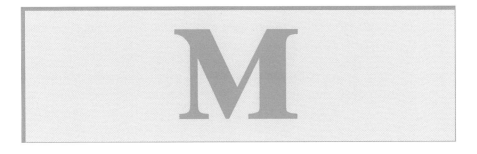

McDonald diagnostic criteria see *Diagnostic criteria, clinical (McDonald).*

McDonald and Halliday diagnostic criteria see *Diagnostic criteria, clinical (McDonald and Halliday).*

Magnetic evoked motor potential (MEP) motor potential evoked by a brief intense magnetic pulse over the scalp. MEP can reveal high rates of central motor conduction time delays in MS.[174,176] In one study of differential sensitivity of techniques for the detection of 'clinically silent' lesions, the SEP was found to be the best, followed by MRI and then MEP.[176]

Magnetic resonance imaging (MRI, NMR) creation of images of objects by use of the nuclear magnetic resonance phenomenon. The immediate practical application involves imaging the distribution of hydrogen nuclei (protons) in the body. The image brightness (or intensity) in a given region is usually dependent (weighted) jointly on the spin density and the relaxation times, with their relative importance determined by the particular imaging technique employed. MRI plays a pivotal role in the diagnosis and prognosis[199] of MS and has become established as the most important surrogate tool for monitoring treatment efficacy in MS—routinely incorporated in both phase II and phase III studies.[3,567] [See also *MRI diagnostic criteria*.]

Magnetic resonance spectroscopy (MRS) use of magnetic resonance to obtain spectral information in the form of peaks that are analysed according to their frequency or chemical shift, peak amplitude and area under the peak. This method allows in vivo measurement of specific changes of metabolite concentrations providing an indication of myelin breakdown as well as a quantifiable index of axonal dysfunction or loss in MS.[537] Reduction of *N*-acetyl aspartate (NAA), a sensitive marker of neuronal damage as well as irreversible neuronal volume loss,[98] has been reported in the lesions and normal-appearing white-matter of MS.[98,99,538] Reduction of NAA on spectroscopy has been correlated with EDSS.[98]

Magnetization prepared rapid acquisition gradient echo (MP-RAGE) three-dimensional and high-resolution MRI sequence that produces T_1-weighted images with very thin slices.[539] The 3D image can be reconstructed in any plane and different section thickness, thus allowing a more complete evaluation of T_1-lesion load and atrophy in MS. MP-RAGE increases the detection rate of T_1-hypointense and enhancing lesions and reduces imprecision due to repositioning errors.[540,541]

Magnetization transfer imaging (MTI) MRI technique based on the exchange of magnetization between a pool of free water and macromolecule-bound water protons. Due to these exchanges, the reduced magnetization of the macromolecular proton pool, which is achieved by application of a saturation radio frequency pulse, is transferred to the free water pool.[542] This MT process may be quantified by comparing the signal intensity of an image with and without an MT saturation pulse. The amount of MT is expressed as magnetization transfer ratio.[542] Myelin is the most complex macromolecular structure in normal white matter and the extent of demyelination in MS may be quantified by measuring MT ratio. Studies in MS patients have demonstrated a decrease in the MT ratio with oedema, demyelination, Wallerian degeneration, axonal injury, gliosis and atrophy.[543-545] Brain histograms of MT ratio have been significantly correlated to EDSS,[546] cognitive deficits[547] and brain atrophy[544] and may be useful in evaluating the natural history and response to therapy in MS treatment trials.[545] [See also *Normal-appearing white matter.*]

Magnetization transfer ratio   see *Magnetization transfer imaging.*

Major histocompatibility complex (MHC)   cluster of genes whose products are associated with cellular recognition and 'self/not self' discrimination. [See *Figure 16.*] The MHC is referred to as the H-2 complex in mice, and the human leukocyte antigens (HLAs) in humans. The MHC loci encode two major classes of membrane molecules, class I and class II MHC molecules that are involved in the interactions with T cells. T-helper cells generally recognize antigens associated with a class II molecule, whereas T-cytotoxic cells generally recognize antigens associated with class I molecules. Several lines of evidence suggest a key role for class II MHC in inflammatory demyelinating diseases.[66,142] [See also *Human leukocyte antigen.*]

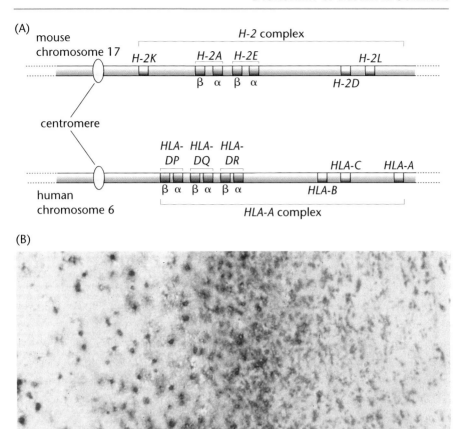

Figure 16   **Major histocompatibility complex:** A: simplified schematic representation of the *H-2* and *HLA* gene complexes. Reproduced with permission.[21A] B: Expression of MHC class II DR in an active MS plaque on macrophages in the plaque on the left and the plaque border in the centre, and on activated microglia in white matter on the right. Immunocytochemical staining with anti-DR antibody, magnification ×110. *(Courtesy of Dr J Newcombe, Institute of Neurology, London.)*

Malignant MS   MS with a rapidly progressive course, leading to significant disability in multiple neurological systems or death a relatively short time after disease onset.[127]

Marburg variant acute fulminant form of MS with rapid progression to death without remission within a few weeks of onset. Pathologically, lesions are more destructive than those usually seen in chronic MS and appear to have occurred simultaneously rather than at different stages. The lesions are, however, histologically similar to the acute MS lesion found in classical MS.[180] The underlying processes that result in this fulminant form are obscure.[290]

Marcus–Gunn pupil see *Afferent pupillary defect*.

MBP gene see *Myelin basic protein gene*.

Methotrexate nonspecific, immunosuppressive and anti-inflammatory agent. Small phase II studies of low-dose oral methotrexate have been reported to be effective in reducing exacerbation rates,[548] and progression of chronic progressive MS,[549] improving neuropsychological function[550] and decreasing lesion load on MRI.[551] There have been no phase III trials to date.

Methylprednisolone powerful steroid introduced as a high-dose, pulsed intravenous infusion which significantly reduces the duration of relapses. [See *Corticosteroids or glucocorticosteroids*.]

Migration alters the risk of MS, suggesting a significant environmental factor. Young immigrants tend to acquire the level of risk of MS associated with their new place of residence. If migration occurs before the age of about 12 to 15 years the risk reduces on moving from a high- to a low-risk area,[336] or increases from a low- to a high-risk area.[337,338] The risk acquired in childhood is not altered by migration during adult years. The evidence that migration from a low- to a high-risk area increases the risk of MS is inconsistent, with high prevalence found in north African migrants to France[337] and in the descendants of African, Asian and West Indian immigrants to the UK.[338] However, Japanese and other immigrants from Asia retain their low susceptibility after migrating to the USA.[552] [See *Figure 17*.]

Minimal Record of Disability (MRD) method to assess handicap and disability for patients with MS. It uses the Incapacity Status Scale (ISS) and Environmental Status Scale (ESS) to supplement the EDSS and its component functional system scales.[313] [See *Incapacity Status Scale* and *Environmental Status Scale*.]

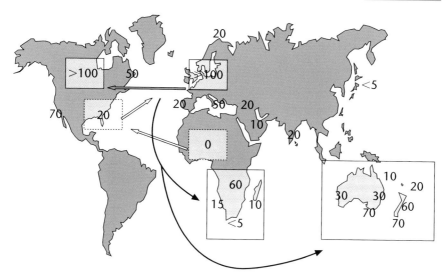

Figure 17 **Migration:** Summary of epidemiological patterns in MS. Reproduced with permission.[644]

Misoprostol   long-acting prostaglandin E analogue that reduces pain by inhibition or excitation of an inhibitory pathway. It is effective in the relief of trigeminal neuralgia in MS.[554]

Mitochondrial DNA (mtDNA)   circular, double-stranded DNA within mitochondria that encodes 13 mitochondrial proteins, transfer RNAs and ribosomal RNAs. Genes necessary for mitochondrial enzymes are often located on the chromosomes of nuclear DNA.[555] Despite the association of Leber's hereditary optic neuropathy and an MS-like illness with mtDNA mutations,[511,556] it is considered unlikely that a susceptibility gene for MS is encoded within the mitochondrial genome.[557] However, there are more than 50 nuclear genes involved in mitochondrial function.

Mitoxantrone (Novantrone)   immunosuppressant of both cellular and humoral components with possible antiviral activity. It exerts an immunosuppressive effect on CD4-helper and cytotoxic T-cells, B lymphocytes and macrophages. Mitoxantrone is able to reduce the annual relapse rate and improve or stabilize RR and/or SP MS patients as assessed by a number of clinical scores. Three controlled trials have demonstrated its efficacy on clinical and MRI criteria *(Table 21)*. A striking reduction in the number of gadolinium-enhancing lesions has been a consistent finding after treatment.[558–561] Due to severe cardiotoxicity (related to total cumulative dose),

103

Table 21 Mitoxantrone and multiple sclerosis—reduction of clinical and MRI activity in controlled trials

	French study[559]	Italian study[563]	MIMS[560,561]
Clinical form of MS	Very active MS; RP or SP	RR	RR or SP
Treatment	20 mg/month for 6 months	8 mg/m² per month for 12 months	12 mg/m² per 3 months for 24 months
Duration of follow-up (months)	6	24	24
Reduction in relapses (%)	77	60	60
Reduction of clinical progression (% of patients with ≥1 point EDSS increase)	84	79	64
Reduction in the number of new MRI lesions (%)	84	52	88
Reduction of active MRI lesions (%)	86	-	86

RP = relapsing-progressive. Adapted with permission.[562]

the duration of therapy is limited and mitoxantrone is only used in selected patients with frequent and disabling exacerbations and/or rapidly progressing disability, or in patients who do not respond to immunomodulatory treatment.[562]

Monozygotic twins   identical twins developing from the same fertilized egg and sharing 100% of their genes. Such twins can differ in a number of ways, including macrochromosomal accidents such as deletions or translocations and the relatively random process of X inactivation in female pairs.

Mortality rate (of MS)   number of individuals dying with MS in the at-risk population in a defined area over a given period. It does not document individuals with MS as a proportion of those who died in the population at that time, but refers to the entire population who could die. More importantly, it can either identify the number of patients dying from MS or the number dying with MS. It is a poor statistic for evaluating the epidemiology of MS.[434]

Motor evoked potential (MEP)   muscle response to electrical stimulation of the cerebral cortex and spinal cord used to study conduction in motor pathways.[564] Central motor conduction times may be markedly prolonged in MS.[565] For patients with SP MS, the frequency of MEP abnormalities is close to 100%.[543] The clinical applicability of the technique has been greatly improved with the advent of magnetic cortical stimulation. [See *Magnetic evoked motor potential*.]

MRI diagnostic criteria   MRI provides a sensitive paraclinical method for detecting disseminated white matter lesions. The abnormalities themselves are nonspecific and diagnostic criteria have been developed to improve specificity (*Table 22*). The criteria focus on the number of hyperintense areas and features such as location, size and activity (gadolinium-enhancing lesion) to significantly improve diagnostic accuracy.

MRI diagnostic criteria (of Barkhof)   the importance of several individual brain MRI criteria at first presentation was evaluated to predict the conversion to CD MS in three groups of patients with clinically isolated syndromes suggestive of MS.[118] The criteria included the optimum cut-off point (number of lesions), one for gadolinium enhancement and juxtacortical lesions, three for periventricular lesions, and nine for the total number of T_2-lesions. The

Table 22 Diagnostic MRI criteria for multiple sclerosis

Reference	Definition	Study design	Sensitivity (%)	Specificity (%)
566	≥4 lesions, or 3 lesions, of which 1 is periventricular	Prospective, at first presentation	94	57
393	≥3 lesions; 2 with the properties: (a) an infratentorial lesion (b) a periventricular lesion (c) a lesion >6 mm	Retrospective, in established MS and controls with white matter lesions(s) on MRI	88	100
118	The optimum number of lesion is: (a) 1 for gadolinium-enhancement (b) 1 for juxtacortical lesion (c) 3 for periventricular lesions (d) 9 for the total number of T_2-lesions	Prospective, at first presentation	61 73 73 73	80 66 73 80
241	Any lesion at the callosal–septal interface	Prospective, in established MS and patients with white matter lesion(s) on MRI	93	98
568	≥1 enhancing lesion and ≥1 nonenhancing lesion	Prospective, at first presentation	59	80
275	Oval shaped T_2-lesions with major axis perpendicular to the ventricular wall	Retrospective, in established MS with abnormal MRI	86	NA

NA = not applicable.

criteria showed higher specificity than those of Paty[566] and Fazekas[393] in predicting the development of MS in patients with clinically isolated clinical syndromes. [See *Table 22.*]

MRI diagnostic criteria (of Fazekas) criteria based on a retrospective review of MRI from asymptomatic volunteers and clinically diagnosed MS patients.[393] The criteria require at least three T_2-lesions and two of the following properties: lesions abutting the body of the lateral ventricles, an infratentorial lesion location and lesion size ≥ 6 mm. The criteria showed both high sensitivity and high specificity in a retrospective study of patients with established MS,[394] but performed less well in a prospective fashion when applied to patients presenting with a clinically isolated syndrome suggestive of MS.[538] [See *Table 22.*]

MRI diagnostic criteria (of McDonald) new MRI diagnostic criteria derived from recent studies[118,193] and recommended by the International Panel on the Diagnosis of Multiple Sclerosis.[192] A diagnosis of MS requires evidence of at least three of the following: (a) one gadolinium-enhancing lesion, or nine T_2 hyperintense lesions if gadolinium-enhancing lesions are not present; (b) at least one infratentorial lesion; (c) at least one juxtacortical lesion (i.e. involving the subcortical U-fibres); (d) at least three periventricular lesions. Lesions should be larger than 3 mm in cross-section. [See *Table 22.*]

MRI diagnostic criteria (of Paty) criteria established from a prospective study that require the presence of four or more T_2-lesions, or three or more T_2-lesions with one lesion bordering the lateral ventricles (periventricular lesion) for the images to be considered 'strongly suggestive' of MS.[566] [See *Table 22.*]

MSCRG (Avonex®, Biogen) phase III trial that enrolled 301 patients treated with placebo vs 30 µg of IFNβ-1a once weekly by intramuscular injection for two years.[331] This trial was terminated prematurely. Active treatment reduced attacks by 18% in all patients in the study. However, in those subjects who completed two years' follow-up, the reduction in the relapse rate was 32%. There was an apparent effect on progression of disability. The primary outcome variable was time to sustained disability progression of at least 1.0 point on the EDSS. The proportion of patients progressing by the end of two years was 34.9% in the placebo group and 21.9% in the INFβ-1a-treated group. However, the number of erroneous progressors in this study was probably high,[569] indicating that some of the benefits may have been due to effects on transient, rather than fixed disability progression. In addition, there was no significant effect on BOD at two years.[570] An effect on reduction of brain atrophy has also been noted.[571] [See *CHAMPS* and *Interferon beta*.]

MS Functional Composite (MSFC) quantitative functional measure of three key clinical dimensions of MS. The tests include assessment of lower limb function by a timed walk of 25 feet,[572] arm/hand function by the Nine-Hole Peg Test,[146] and cognitive function by the three-second version of the Paced Auditory Serial Addition Test (PASAT).[232] Scores are converted to standard scores (z-scores), which are then averaged to form a single MSFC score. The MSFC provides a relatively balanced assessment of the impact of MS on diverse clinical dimensions of MS and has proved to be sensitive, valid and optimal for MS clinical outcome measures.[573–575] MSFC scores have been found to correlate with EDSS,[311,575] MRI lesion load[576] and self-reported quality of life.[577] Furthermore, baseline MSFC scores and change in MSFC score correlate with both disability status and the severity of whole brain atrophy[578] and cognitive function.[579] A detailed administration and scoring manual is available.[580] [See *Appendix 4*.]

MS Quality of Life Instrument (MSQOL-54) QoL tool derived from Short Form-36 [see *Appendix 6*] that evaluates general health perceptions, social functions, change in health status, health distress, overall quality of life, pain, fatigue, sexual function and satisfaction, and cognitive function.[581] It has been reported to have an acceptable degree of reliability and construct validity and is useful as a supplementary outcome measure in phase III clinical trials.[365] Quality of life as measured by MSQOL-54 is reported to relate in part to brain hypointense lesions and atrophy shown on MRI and to the scores of the EDSS.[582] [See *Appendix 8*.]

MS Quality of Life Inventory (MSQLI) tool that employs widely-used generic health-related QoL and established symptom-specific measures for fatigue, pain/disturbing sensations, sexual function, bladder function, bowel function, perceived visual function, emotional status and social functioning. Objective measures of impairment (EDSS, quantitative measures of upper and lower limb function, visual acuity, a brief neuropsychological battery) and handicap are included. This measure is integrated into the WHO classification schema for impairment, disability and handicap effects of MS on an individual's life.[583] Although the instrument has acceptable psychometric properties and is applicable to patients with varied MS symptoms, its responsiveness has not been established.[583]

MtDNA   see *Mitochondrial DNA*.

Multimodality evoked potentials   term generally used to describe combination of EP recordings in three modalities (VEP, SEP, BAEP). Multimodality EP testing has been reported to be slightly more sensitive than MRI in several studies.[150,584,585] In 222 MS patients followed for $2\frac{1}{2}$ years, multimodality EPs and MRI were found to be equally effective for predicting which patients would be diagnosed as MS or have a deteriorating clinical course.[586]

Multiple sclerosis (MS, demyelinating disease, disseminated sclerosis) generally considered to be a primarily demyelinating T-cell-mediated chronic inflammatory disease of the CNS in which an autoimmune response to myelin proteins of the CNS is triggered by one or more exogenous agents in a genetically susceptible host. Clinical manifestations typically appear between 20 and 40 years of age with focal, multifocal, episodic or persisting neurological symptoms and signs.

Multiplicity of (separate) lesions   to be certain of the presence of multiple lesions, in order to satisfy diagnostic criteria for 'dissemination in space', symptoms must not be explicable on the basis of pathology at a single anatomical site. For example, simultaneously occurring internuclear ophthalmoplegia, facial weakness and corticospinal signs could all be due to a single brainstem lesion and thus cannot be used as evidence of more than one lesion. Optic neuritis involving both eyes simultaneously, or with involvement of the second eye within 30 days of the first (provided that compression of the chiasm by tumour or aneurysm has been ruled out), would be considered due to a single lesion. Only lesions that involve distinctly different parts of the CNS can be attributed to separate lesions.[191]

Multiscale Depression Inventory   measure comprised of separate scales for mood, evaluative and vegetative symptoms.[587] It is recommended for recording cognitive and psychological function in MS databases.[239]

Mutation   change in the sequence of DNA at a genetic locus.

Myelin   lipid-rich protein membrane enclosing and effectively insulating axons in the white matter of the central and peripheral nervous system to ensure the propagation of impulses by saltatory conduction. It is the major structural component of normal white matter and accounts for about 25% of the dry weight of the brain.[588] The antigenic structure of myelin, which includes the epitopes myelin basic protein (MBP), proteolipid protein (PLP) and myelin–oligodendrocyte glycoprotein (MOG), renders the CNS potentially vulnerable to autoimmune-mediated processes. However, the nature of any putative auto-antigen in MS remains to be elucidated.[441,589] [See also *Autoantigen, Myelin associated glycoprotein, Myelin basic protein, Myelin proteolipid protein* and *Oral myelin.*]

Myelin-associated glycoprotein (MAG)   minor component (about 1%) of total CNS protein. Also present in peripheral nervous system myelin. Considered a potential autoantigen in demyelinating disease.[589] T cells specific for MAG have been reported in the Lewis rat.[590,591] MAG-reactive CD4+ T cells and anti-MAG antibodies have been demonstrated in the peripheral blood and CSF in MS.[445,592] MAG IgM antibodies are associated with a demyelinating peripheral neuropathy.

Myelin basic protein (MBP)   protein of the myelin sheath that comprises 30% of CNS myelin protein. The presence of MBP or its fragments in CSF can be used as an index of active demyelination and a surrogate marker of disease activity.[593,594] CSF MBP levels in active MS patients are increased and have been correlated with relapse rate and the number of gadolinium-enhanced lesions on MRI.[594] CSF MBP levels have also been found to correlate with visual acuity in optic neuritis (ON) and EDSS in MS patients.[217,595] Autoantibodies directed against MBP[596,597] may or may not have a direct pathogenic role. By contrast, MOG specific autoantibodies may mediate demyelination.[598,599] [See also *Myelin oligodendrocyte glycoprotein.*]

Myelin basic protein gene (MBP gene)   gene encoded on chromosome 18 which has been linked to MS susceptibility in Finnish,[600] but not Swedish[601] or Italian families.[602] [See also *Myelin basic protein.*]

Myelin basic protein-like material (MBPLM)   material that reacts with antibodies to MBP.[603] The levels of MBPLM in CSF are related to both the mass of CNS myelin damage and how recently the damage occurred.[604] Urinary MBPLM does not reflect acute disease activity in MS, but correlates with the disease burden on MRI. Increased levels may antedate the clinical transition from a relapsing–remitting to a chronic progressive course.[605,606]

Myelinoclastic diffuse sclerosis   see *Schilder's disease*.

Myelin oligodendrocyte glycoprotein (MOG) minor component of myelin proteins exclusively expressed at the outer surface of myelin sheaths and oligodendrocytes.[607] A single Ig V-like domain exposed at the membrane surface represents the target for an antibody that can cause experimental demyelination[608–610] resembling MS.[440,611] Enhanced responses of T cells and B cells to MOG have been reported in the peripheral blood and CSF of MS patients[598,599] and early and persistent anti-MOG-Ig antibody responses are found in patients with MS.[441] Anti-MOG antibodies enhance pathology in EAE. The possibility that MOG is a primary target of the humoral autoimmune process in MS needs further investigation.[441,599]

Myelin proteolipid protein (PLP)   major component (about 50%) of myelin protein thought to be a candidate autoantigen in MS.[443] PLP autoantibody and PLP-reactive T cells are present in the blood and CSF of MS patients.[443,444,598] Human in vitro studies have failed to demonstrate PLP antibody-mediated demyelination,[612,613] but EAE can be induced by PLP, and PLP-reactive T cells can transfer EAE.[614]

Myelopathy   pathological condition of the spinal cord. Symptoms and signs depend on the specific tract involvement and severity. Acute spinal cord lesions in MS are often partial or incomplete [see *Acute (subacute) myelopathy* and *Transverse myelitis*].

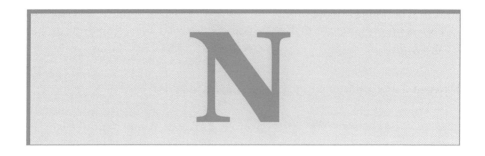

N20 one of the principal wavepeaks or potentials of the median SEP. It arises from the postcentral primary somatosensory cortex and has been found to be useful for detecting abnormalities in the major sensory pathways and for serial SEP studies in MS.[148,362] [See also *Somatosensory evoked potential.*]

***N*-acetyl aspartate (NAA)** brain metabolite that is exclusively present in neurons and axons and is therefore used as an in vivo marker for neuro-axonal loss and as an index for neuronal viability or function.[615] [See also *Magnetic resonance spectroscopy.*]

Natalizumab see *Anti-α 4 integrin antibody.*

Neopterin product of IFN-γ activated macrophages that is an indirect measure of both the levels of IFN-γ and IFN-induced macrophage activity.[616] Elevated levels of neopterin have been found in the CSF[617,618] and serum[617] in MS. An association between urinary neopterin levels and MS disease activity has been reported.[619]

Neuroantigen nervous system auto antigen, examples include: *Myelin basic protein, Myelin proteolipid protein* and *Myelin oligodendrocyte glycoprotein* in the central nervous system and P2 protein in the peripheral nervous system.

Neurofilament protein major structural protein of neurons that maintains the size, shape and calibre of the axon. Increased concentrations of neuro-filament protein in CSF are found during clinical exacerbations and may be a marker of axonal damage in MS.[620]

Neuromyelitis optica see *Devic's neuromyelitis optica.*

New active lesion   new active lesions on MRI are defined as newly enhancing lesions on T_1 images, or new or enlarging lesions on T_2-weighted images [see also *Active lesion*].

Newly enhancing T_1 lesions   currently enhancing lesions on MRI after gadolinium injection.

Nine-Hole Peg Test (9-HPT)   quantitative method for assessing disability of the upper limb,[146] which is one component of the MSFC.[573] Patients insert pegs one by one into each of nine holes laid out in a square pattern, and then remove the pegs one by one. Each hand is tested twice. The time taken to insert and remove all the pegs is recorded. The method is sensitive, reliable and easily applied.[146] [See *Appendix 4.*]

Nitric oxide (NO)   inorganic gas and free radical that mediates a variety of biological functions, including neurotransmission, vasodilatation and cytotoxicity.[621] In vitro studies have implicated the free radical NO in oligodendrocyte death.[622,623] Increased levels of NO metabolites, nitrate and nitrite, are found in the CSF[624,625] and serum of patients with MS.[625,626] As NO and its derivative peroxynitrite are cytotoxic to both oligodendrocytes and neurons, they are potential mediators of demyelination and axonal loss in MS.[625]

Node of Ranvier   constriction occurring on myelinated nerve fibres at regular intervals of about 1 mm where the myelin sheath is absent and the axon is enclosed only by Schwann cell processes.

Normal appearing white matter (NAWM)   areas of macroscopically normal white matter with normal signal intensity on conventional PD/T_2 and T_1 MRI scans that occur around and between obvious MS plaques. Histopathological studies have demonstrated widespread discrete abnormalities in the NAWM.[627] MRI investigations using T_1 and T_2 magnetization decay curves, spectroscopy, MTI and diffusion tensor imaging have provided evidence of widespread axonal damage or loss in NAWM of MS.[97,99,538,628–630] These changes may be attributed to microscopic lesions and/or Wallerian degeneration in the absence of overt inflammation.[631,632]

Novantrone   see *Mitoxantrone*.

Numbers needed to treat (NNT) measure to determine the impact of a treatment compared with a population at risk or a placebo group, to prevent an adverse event. Statistically it is the reciprocal of absolute risk reduction of a treatment. Therefore, NNT = $1/(pC - pT)$, where pC = proportion of control with an adverse event, and pT = proportion of treatment group with an adverse event.

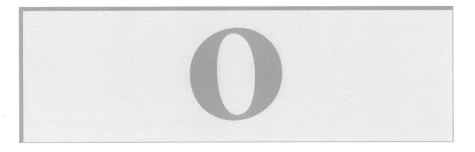

OKT3 see *Anti-CD3*.

Oligoclonal bands (OCBs) abnormal immunoglobulins in the CSF. Isoelectric focusing is the most sensitive method of detection[195,633] and their presence, although nonspecific, supports the diagnosis.[191] Although found in more than 95% of patients with CD MS,[195,633] they may also be present in many other neurological diseases. [See also *Intrathecal IgG synthesis* and *Laboratory support*.]

Oligodendrocyte (OG) myelin-forming cell of the CNS that is responsible for the elaboration and maintenance of myelin in the CNS. [See *Figure 18*.] Destruction of OGs has been considered to be a primary cause of demyelination.[94] Oligodendrocyte loss and the failure of the OG precursor population to expand and generate new oligodendrocytes may account for the failure of myelin repair in chronic MS.[184] It is well accepted that OGs are largely absent from chronic MS lesions.[182–184] When high numbers of OGs are present, rapid and complete remyelination may occur in the early stages of an active lesion.[517,634,635] OGs initially respond to a demyelinating insult by proliferating and elaborating new myelin, but the cells are eventually lost.[636] The mechanisms that underlie oligodendrocyte death may include cytokines,[637] activation of cell death signals,[638] the free radical nitric oxide[623] and apoptosis.[639] [See also *Dying-back oligodendrogliopathy*.]

Oligodendrocyte progenitor cells (OPCs) cells that can develop into new, fully differentiated oligodendrocytes capable of regenerating and maintaining myelin.[640] Significant numbers of OPCs may be present in the centre of new demyelinating lesions, apparently unaffected by the inflammatory destructive processes,[635,640,641] but they are rare in chronic MS lesions.[184] The failure of the OPCs to expand and generate new oligodendrocytes may be responsible for the failure of myelin repair in the later stages of the disease.[184]

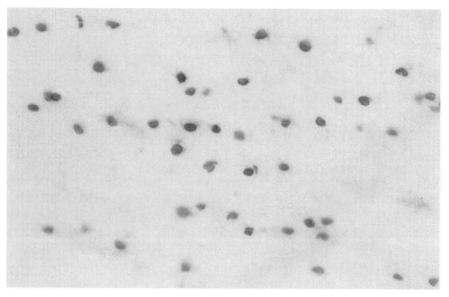

(A)

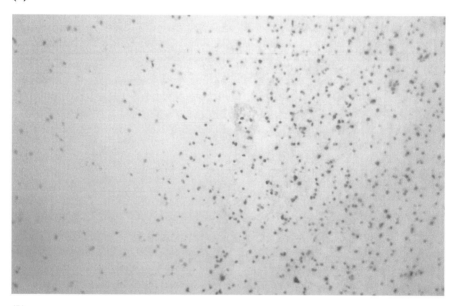

(B)

Figure 18 **Oligodendrocytes:** A: Oligodendrocytes in normal control brain white matter, magnification ×440. B: Chronic plaque with loss of oligodendrocytes on the left and white matter with normal numbers of oligodendrocytes on the right. Immunocytochemical staining with antibody directed against the 14E antigen, magnification ×110. *(Courtesy of Dr J Newcombe, Institute of Neurology, London.)*

Ondansetron   specific (5HT$_3$) serotonin antagonist reported to be effective in treating cerebellar tremor.[642]

Onset   see *Disease onset.*

Onset symptoms   first symptoms that can be attributed definitely to MS. *Table 23* lists first symptoms that are (a) acceptable, with caveats to date of first onset for epidemiological purposes and (b) possibly acceptable, with caveats.

Table 23 Onset symptoms
(a)   *Definite: these symptoms must last for at least 24 hours:*
Unilateral optic/retrobulbar neuritis
Acquired monocular colour blindness
Oscillopsia
True binocular diplopia
Tic douloureux (under age 40)
Hemifacial spasm (under age 40)
Acute unilateral diminution of hearing (under age 40)
Transient acute nonpositional vertigo (under age 40)
Transient scanning speech
Transverse myelitis
Lhermitte's symptom
Gait ataxia
Unilateral dysmetria/intention tremor/incoordination
Sensory useless hand syndrome
Transient weakness/paraesthesias of one entire limb
Transient painless urinary retention (under age 40)
Transient painless urinary urgency/incontinence in men (under age 40)
(b)   *Possible: in order for these symptoms to be used as onset markers, they must be followed by a definite symptom within two years:*
Unilateral facial palsy
Transient painless urinary frequency in men (under age 40)
Transient hemiparesis (under age 40)
Organic erectile dysfunction
Painful tonic seizures
Adapted with permission.[320]

Onset-adjusted prevalence rate (OAPR)   number of cases including symptomatic MS within the specified population at a point in time.[201] Measure is
based on a well-defined, ethnically homogeneous population who have
spent the critical years of putative acquisition of the disease (i.e. between the
ages of 5 and 15 years, or puberty) in the geographical area under study. It
may, more precisely, determine the role of genetic susceptibility and potentially significant environmental factors affecting disease acquisition.[201]

Optic neuritis (ON) (retrobulbar neuritis, RBN)   disturbance of visual function involving reduction or loss of vision (typically unilateral, but sometimes
bilateral), of abrupt or gradual onset which may then worsen over hours,
days or weeks, due to an inflammatory lesion in the optic nerve. Visual loss
may be total or partial and usually preferentially involves the central field.
Associated features include retro-orbital pain on eye movement in about
53–92% of cases,[24,643] central scotoma, afferent pupillary defect and loss of
colour vision. Pain on eye movement, attributed to stretching of the
meninges around a swollen optic nerve,[24] may precede the onset of visual
symptoms in 39% of episodes.[643] Average duration is 4 to 6 weeks with
gradual recovery in most cases (little or no recovery in about 15%). ON is the
presenting symptom in about 25% of patients with MS[644] and over 50% of
cases subsequently develop CD MS.[645–650] An abnormal MRI at the time of
ON is significantly associated with an increased risk of subsequent CD
MS.[14,199,331,651,652]

Optic papillopathy (papillitis)   swollen optic nerve head or optic disc (as
seen on ophthalmoscopy). This occurs in 20–30% of patients with ON[24,643]
due to an inflammatory lesion situated close to the nerve head (in most ON
the optic disc appearance is normal because the lesion is retrobulbar). A
variety of other conditions can cause optic papillopathy, including
ischaemic pathologies.

Oral myelin   oral administration of myelin induces immune tolerance by sup-
pressing systemic T-cell-mediated immune responses.[653] No treatment efficacy was demonstrated in a phase III study of oral myelin.[654,655]

Oscillopsia   illusory movement of the environment caused by images of sta-
tionary objects moving across the retina. It is often associated with nystagmus in MS, usually due to lesions in the vestibulocerebellar connections, or
medial longitudinal fasciculus (vertical oscillopsia).

Outcome measure parameter used to show a difference in outcome between the placebo and active treatment arms in a therapeutic trial (see *Table 16*). Outcome measures in MS trials may be clinical (relapse rate or the proportion of relapse-free patients), EDSS, hospitalization or paraclinical tests (MRI outcome, CSF analysis) [see also *Endpoint* and *Table 16*].

Ovoid lesion oval-shaped, hyperintense areas in white matter oriented perpendicular to the ventricles on axial T_2-weighted MRI [see *Figure 19*]. They are regarded as one of the two patterns of white matter disease that are relatively specific for MS.[275] [See also *Dawson's finger* and *Periventricular lesions*.]

OWIMS (Rebif®, Serono International SA) phase II/III treatment trial that investigated the effects of once-weekly subcutaneous injections of two doses (22 μg and 44 μg) of IFNβ-1a on monthly MRI for 48 weeks. The high-dose (44 μg), but not the low-dose (22 μg) treatment resulted in a 53% reduction in the number of combined active MRI lesions.[656] The proportion of active MRI scans was reduced by 5% (versus placebo) by 22 μg weekly, and by 17% by 44 μg. There was a mean reduction of 19% in the relapse rate in patients treated with 44 μg weekly. [See also *Interferon beta-1a*.]

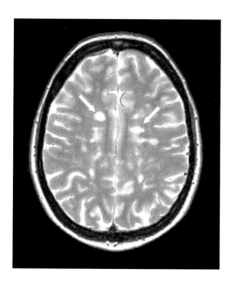 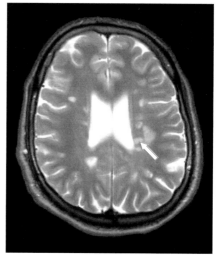

Figure 19 Ovoid lesions: Axial T_2-weighted images in clinically definite multiple scerosis. Arrows indicate typical ovoid lesions in periventricular white matter.

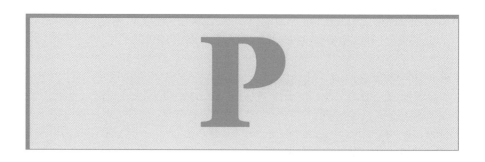

P100 designation of the major positive wave (or potential) in VEP recordings. The VEP is a compound response made up of many different potentials, but the P100 is most often used for clinical latency and amplitude measurements. Its mean latency is approximately 100 ms after pattern reversal, but varies with stimulus-related variables (contrast, check size, luminance), recording factors (electrode position) and subject variables (age, gender, refraction, etc.), so normal limits must be established for each laboratory [see also *Visual evoked potential*].

Paced Auditory Serial Addition Test (PASAT) measure of cognitive function that assesses auditory information processing speed and flexibility, as well as calculation ability.[232] Changes in performance on the PASAT correlate significantly with changes in total lesion volume on MRI.[657] There are several versions; the 2-second and 3-second versions are used in the Brief Repeatable Battery, but only the 3-second version in the MSFC [see *Appendix 4*].

Pain acute or chronic pain is reported by 65% of MS patients at sometime during their illness.[658] Chronic pain is often referred to the extremities or back and the frequency increases with advanced age and disease duration.[323,658] In many cases pain is caused by the secondary disability, i.e. an abnormal posture, and not the underlying disease process. Acute pain due to optic neuritis is most frequent (50%), followed by Lhermitte's sign (30%) and trigeminal neuralgia.[526,658] Tonic seizures and flexor spasms due to advanced spasticity are often painful.

Pain rating scales methods of measuring pain in MS are mostly not disease-specific techniques. A simple ordinal scale may be used and the severity of pain rated from 1 to 10 (10 being most severe). Linear scales require the patient to position a mark on a line to indicate an existing level of pain. The

McGill pain questionnaire has also been used in MS and is appropriate for therapeutic trials directed specifically toward the treatment of pain.[365,659].

Paraclinical (diagnostic) evidence   demonstration, by means of various tests and procedures, of the existence of a 'clinically silent' lesion in the CNS, which is not causing signs of neurological dysfunction, but may or may not have caused neurological symptoms in the past.[191] Such tests include hot bath test, evoked response studies, neuroimaging procedures and urological assessment, provided that these tests and procedures follow the guidelines and are interpreted according to the established criteria.[191] Today, only evoked potentials and neuroimaging are generally accepted methods for paraclinical demonstration of lesions in the CNS.

Paroxysmal syndromes   brief episodic, often frequent and repeated, stereotyped symptoms, that are generally triggered by movement or sensory stimuli. Most arise in brain stem or spinal cord and their nature depends on the site of origin.[662] The most frequent are trigeminal neuralgia, tonic spasms, dysarthria, ataxia, paraesthesiae, itching, diplopia and akinesia. The pathophysiological mechanism is considered to be due to a transverse ephaptic current spreading across partially demyelinated fibre tracts.[663] They usually respond well to membrane-stabilizing drugs such as carbamazepine, phenytoin, gabapentin or misoprostol.[400,554,665,666] [See also *Specific symptoms e.g. Akynesia, Ataxia, Diplopia, Dysarthria, Itching, etc.*]

Participation (WHO definition)   nature and extent of a person's involvement in life situations resulting from the interaction of impairments and limitations in activities on the one hand, and the context in which a person lives, on the other. Contextual factors include environmental and personal factors that constitute the complete context of an individual's life.[5] [See also *Activity limitation.*]

Pattern reversal   standard visual stimulus used in recording diagnostic visual evoked potentials (VEPs). It is usually generated by a video display attached to a pattern generator or video card connected to a computer. The checks on a black and white checkerboard pattern reverse from black to white (or vice versa) at a rate of about 2 Hz. The latency of the response can be affected by the pattern luminance, sharpness of focus, contrast and check size.

Paty diagnostic criteria (MRI)   see *MRI diagnostic criteria (of Paty).*

Pemoline synthetic organic chemical that acts as a cerebral stimulant and has been reported to ameliorate MS-associated fatigue in open-label pilot studies[667] and one double-blind, placebo-controlled trial.[668] Side-effects include irritability, insomnia, dizziness, anorexia, nausea and headache.

Pentoxifylline phosphodiesterase inhibitor that has been reported to reduce the production of TNF-α in some,[669] but not all studies.[670,671] Pentoxifylline therapy confers no direct benefits for MS patients,[671] but may reduce early side effects of IFNβ-1b treatment.[672]

Periphlebitis retina (perivenous sheathing) areas of fluffy white exudative lesions surrounding the retinal veins seen during optic neuritis or in MS. Acute periphlebitis retina is characterized by lymphocytic cuffing and occasional haemorrhagic exudates, while chronic lesions show a scanty infiltration of plasma cells and thick laminated collagenous repair.[673] The reported prevalence of periphlebitis retina in MS has varied from 10 to 20%.[673]

Perivenous sheathing see *Periphlebitis retina*.

Periventricular lesions hyperintense areas adjacent to the ventricles seen particularly on T_2-weighted MRI [see *Figures 13 and 19*]. Lesions may be ovoid and orientated with their long axis at right angles to the ventricle due to the periventricular focus of the pathology, which follows the course of the subependymal veins.[275] Later in the disease the abnormal areas become larger, irregular and confluent.

Persistently enhancing T_1 lesions enhancing lesions that were enhancing on an earlier sequential scan.

Phase I treatment trial trial for the initial phase of testing of a new drug in healthy human volunteers. Phase I studies are designed to determine the metabolism and phamarcological action of a drug in humans, to identify potential adverse events (toxicity) and provide some early evidence of effectiveness.

Phase II treatment trial an exploratory or preliminary clinical trial conducted to define the appropriate dose and regimen for patients with the disease under study. It should provide some information on the clinical effectiveness of therapy versus adverse effects. The primary outcome measure for phase II trials in MS is based on various analyses of enhancing lesions on MRI.[3]

Phase III treatment trial (definitive study)   trial designed to evaluate the overall benefit–risk relationship of a drug and provide substantial evidence of a product's safety and efficacy.

Phase IV treatment trial   postmarketing study conducted to collect and accumulate safety and efficacy data in the context of clinical practice after approval and licensing by regulatory authorities (e.g. FDA).

Phenocopy   phenotypically similar cases of disease that differ in pathogenesis from a known genetic cause. The occurrence of such cases can confound linkage analysis.

Phenotype   observable characteristics of an individual as determined by his/her genotype and the environment in which he/she develops. In a more limited sense, the outward expression of some particular gene or genes. Thus a heterozygote and a homozygote for a fully dominant gene will have the same phenotype, but different genotype.

Phosphenes   brief (1–2 seconds), subjectively perceived, flashes of bright light precipitated by lateral eye movement, highly characteristic of ON either in acute or recovery phase. Best elicited from the affected eye in a dark or dimly lit room with eyes closed.

Plaque   abnormal region of white matter (the hallmark of MS pathology) where demyelination is occurring, or has occurred. It is characterized by variable myelin destruction, gliosis, remyelination and axonal loss. Based on the extent of scarring and inflammatory activity, MS plaques may be acute/recent, chronic, chronic active or shadow plaques.[10]

Plasma cell   terminally differentiated, antibody-producing B cell.

Plasma exchange (PE)   effective means of removing antibodies and other proteins from the circulation. Some studies have shown the beneficial effect of PE in patients with chronic progressive MS,[674–676] but others have been inconclusive.[29,677,678] In a large multicentre, placebo-controlled study, the value of PE could not be proven.[268] A meta-analysis has suggested that PE may be beneficial to patients with chronic progressive MS who are likely to experience neurological decline during the ensuing 12–24 months.[679] Plasma exchange may have a role in treating patients with acute transverse myelitis who have failed to respond to high-dose intravenous glucocortico-steroids.[680]

Plasmapheresis   see *Plasma exchange.*

Polyarteritis nodosa   systemic disease, common in older males, with necrotizing vasculitis of small- and medium-size arteries characterized by episodic infarction or haemorrhage in various organs, notably the kidney.[681] Neurological complications of polyarteritis nodosa tend to be late and evidence of systemic disease, including fever, malaise, weight loss, myalgia and arthralgia, which are not features of MS, is usually present.

Polyunsaturated fatty acid (PFA) diet   a diet rich in PFA may be beneficial for relapse severity and disability progression in early cases.[682,683]

Poser Committee criteria   see *Diagnostic criteria, clinical (Poser).*

Possible MS   classification category for a patient with appropriate clinical presentation who has not yet been evaluated, or whose evaluation meets some, but not all, of the necessary criteria.[192] [See *Diagnostic, clinical criteria.*]

Post hoc cluster analysis   study of an excess number of new cases of a disease within a small area and over a short period. The study provides a means to investigate the cause of an outbreak of the disease in the area. There are several examples of the method applied to MS, including the most studied high-prevalence case material from the Faroe Islands.[343,346,684–690] These studies have failed to establish any causative environmental factors for the acquisition of MS.

Prednisolone   oral steroid sometimes used for treating relapses of MS. It is usually given in a tapering dose, for a period of three weeks or less, due to the side effects and the risk of dependence. Some studies have suggested that the benefits are similar to high-dose intravenous methylprednisolone.[691] [See also *Corticosteroids or glucocorticosteroids.*]

Preliminary treatment trial   see *Phase II treatment trial.*

Prevalence   number of all new and old cases combined, expressed per unit of population within the community at a given point in time.[692,693] Only living patients are counted on the chosen prevalence day. Prevalence rate should include all patients affected by MS, i.e. who had had symptoms of MS and who were subsequently diagnosed, although such a diagnosis might not have been made on prevalence day.[201] An increase in the absolute number of cases identified in different parts of the world since the 1950s[687] has been attributed to improvements in diagnostic methodology. The distribution of MS can be broadly classified into low, medium and high prevalence.[692–694] High-risk ($>30/10^5$) areas include northern Europe, northern USA, Canada, southern Australia and New Zealand; medium-risk ($5–30/10^5$) areas include southern Europe, southern USA and northern Australia; and low-risk ($<5/10^5$) Asia, South America. The direct relationship between the prevalence of MS and latitude in Europe has diminished with the finding of a higher prevalence in Italy than was previously recognized.[695] Genetic factors play an important role in determining prevalence in Europe and USA (e.g. effects of Scandinavian and northern European heritage).[695,696] The effects of latitude on prevalence rates are less complicated in Australia and New Zealand where the population genetics are relatively homogeneous (e.g. little variation in HLA–DR2 distribution).[697] Both environmental influences and genetic susceptibility affect the acquisition of MS.[320,698] [See also *Latitude, effects on prevalence*.]

Primary MS affection (PMSA)   terminology that has been applied in a theory on the acquisition of MS which was developed from epidemiological observations, e.g. single, widespread, specific, systemic infectious disease whose acquisition in virgin populations follows 2 years of exposure starting between age 11 and 45.[699] Only a small proportion of the affected patients develop clinical neurological MS after 6 (virgin) or 12 (endemic) years' incubation after PMSA acquisition. PMSA is transmissible only during part, or all, of this systemic phase that ends before the usual age of clinical MS onset, by which point it has either become sequestered in the CNS or it has disappeared from the individual.

Primary progressive MS (PP MS)   disease course characterized by progressive deterioration from the onset of disease, without clear-cut relapses or remissions, but with occasional plateaux and temporary minor improvements.[127] Approximately 10% to 15% of patients experience progression from onset. This course tends to onset later in life than typical RR MS and the female propensity seen in RR MS is in most series less obvious or absent.[700] Diagnostic criteria for definite, probable and possible PP MS have been recently proposed.[192,701]

Primary progressive MS, definite MS with solely progressive course for at least one year, positive CSF and either positive MRI evidence, or equivocal MRI evidence and a delayed visual evoked potential.[701]

Primary progressive MS, possible patients suspected to have PP MS with clinical progression for at least one year and equivocal MRI evidence or delayed VEP.[701]

Primary progressive MS, probable patients suspected to have PP MS with either (a) clinical progression for at least one year, positive CSF and equivocal MRI evidence, or delayed VEP, or (b) clinical progression for at least one year, positive MRI or equivocal MRI evidence and a delayed VEP (CSF evidence either unavailable or negative).[701]

PRISMS (Rebif®, Serono International SA) a large phase III trial involving 560 RR MS patients who were treated with two doses of IFNβ-1a (22 μg and 44 μg) subcutaneously three times a week for two years. The treatment showed significant efficacy in reducing the number of relapses (−29% on low-dose and −32% on high-dose treatment), delaying disease progression and, reducing disease activity and burden of disease on MRI.[213,333] Further analysis using area under curve confirmed the beneficial effect of IFNβ-1a in higher doses on accumulating disability.[57] These benefits of treatment remained during a 2-year extension of this trial with a significant advantage of high-dose (44 μg) over low-dose (22 μg) and early over late (two years of placebo first) treatment.[460] Neutralizing antibodies to IFNβ-1a appeared several months after starting treatment and the high dose was associated with a lower incidence of NABs than the low dose (24% versus 12.5%).[333] The presence of NABs reduced the efficacy of the treatment on relapses and MRI activity in the third and fourth years of treatment.

Programmed cell death see *Apoptosis*.

Progression index measure of the rate of disease worsening in terms of disability accumulation derived by the difference in EDSS at two time points/time difference.

Progressive–relapsing MS (PR MS)   disease course characterized by progression from onset, with superimposed clear acute relapses, with or without full recovery. The periods between relapses are characterized by continuing progression.[127] Considered a rare clinical course.

Pro-inflammatory cytokines   see *Cytokines*.

Proteolipid protein mRNA   very early marker of oligodendrocyte differentiation that is expressed in cells of the oligodendrocyte lineage during myelination and maintenance of myelin. It is present in demyelinated areas and its expression may be reduced when these cells are under immunological attack.[702]

Proton density   see *Spin density*.

Pruritus   see *Itching*.

Psychosis   delusional state with or without hallucinations, which is not as common as other affective disorders in MS. MRI suggests that affective psychosis may be associated particularly with temporal or periventricular pathology in MS.[704]

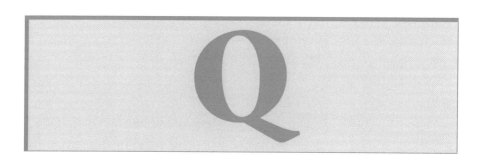

Quality of life (QoL) defined as 'the status of a person as judged by himself/herself in three important domains of life: physical (i.e. self-perceived impairment or disability), psychological (e.g. mostly anxiety, depression and fear) and social functioning (i.e. social support, contacts and role fulfilment). Some QoL instruments used in MS were developed for use in other diseases (e.g. geriatric or chronic disease) and some are 'disease-specific' to MS. MS-specific measures include: the *MS Quality of Life Instrument*,[581] the *Functional Assessment of MS*[397] and the *MS Quality of Life Inventory*[705] [see *Table 24*].

Quantitative Neurological Examination (QNE) battery of tests used to measure cognition, strength, steadiness, reaction, speed, coordination, sensation, fatigue, gait, station and selected skills of daily living.[314] It has been used in some MS trials,[707] but is not widely accepted.

Quinoline-3-carboxamide see *Roquinimex*.

Table 24 Quality of life instruments used in MS

QoL instrument	Reference
General	
Sickness Impact Profile	428
Nottingham Health Profile	429
Short Form Health Survey (SF-36)	430
Specific	
MS Quality of Life (MSQOL)-54 Instrument	581
Disability and Impact Profile	706
Minimal Record of Disability	313
Farmer Quality of Life Index	380
Functional Assessment of MS (FAMS)	397
MS Quality of Life Inventory (MSQLI)	705

R

Race MS is primarily a disease of Caucasians with high incidence in northern Europe, continental North America and Australia. It is much less prevalent in East Asia, the Arabian Peninsula, Africa, continental South America and India.[411,415] Among Caucasians, Scandinavians and their descendants are the most susceptible.[320,708] There are no known cases in ethnically pure Eskimos, Inuits, North and South Amerindians, Australian aborigines, Maoris, Pacific Islanders or Lapps.[320] Race may also have effects on the phenotypic expression of MS, namely clinical manifestation, site of lesions, disease course and prognosis.[62]

Rebif® (Serono International SA) see *Interferon beta-1a*.

Recurrent enhancing T₁-lesions enhancing lesions on MRI that have re-appeared at a site where an earlier lesion had disappeared.

Recurrent T₂-lesions lesion re-appearing on MRI at a site where an earlier lesion had disappeared.[334]

Relapse (attack, episode, exacerbation, bout) clinical expression of an underlying inflammatory episode in the CNS white matter. A relapse, as defined by McAlpine[644] is 'a new symptom, or the re-appearance of a previous symptom at a time after an initial attack'. The requirement for the symptom(s) to last at least 24 hours, at least when evaluating the effect of a treatment, has also been considered necessary.[189] A relapse has been defined, for the purpose of clinical trials, as 'the occurrence of a symptom or symptoms of neurological dysfunction, in the absence of fever, with or without objective confirmation, lasting more than 24 hours'.[191] However, single paroxysmal episodes (e.g. a tonic spasm) are not considered to constitute a relapse, whereas multiple episodes occurring over not less than 24 hours may do.[192] Attacks have been classified as monosymptomatic or polysymptomatic,

mild or severe, 'confirmed' (i.e. associated with clinical signs) or unconfirmed. The average attack duration is from 4 to 6 weeks, but may vary from 1
or 2 days up to many months. Thirty days is agreed to separate the onset of
the first event from the onset of a second event.[192] Relapse rate is significantly
reduced after treatment with IFN-β[333,459] or Copolymer 1.[332]

Relapsing–progressive MS   old term used for secondary progressive MS with
superimposed relapses. This term was abandoned in the classification by
Lublin et al.[127]

Relapsing–remitting MS (RR MS)   disease course characterized by a clear
history of relapses and remissions, either with full recovery or with sequelae
and residual deficit(s) upon recovery. Periods between relapses are characterized by lack of evidence of clinical disease progression,[127] although MRI activity shows that inflammatory disease activity is continuous in most RR MS
patients most of the time and some disease parameters that are not commonly
measured clinically (e.g. brain atrophy, memory and cognive processing) may
be worsening without symptoms. From this point of view, periods of apparent
clinical remission in the RR MS phase can be misleading. Approximately 80%
of patients with MS will start with a relapsing–remitting phase and most of
these will go on eventually to secondary progression. NB: the future course of
RR MS and the time to SP MS in an individual patient is unpredictable,
although MRI changes at the time of diagnosis have some prognostic value.

Relative risk   risk conferred by a characteristic (e.g. race, gender, HLA DR2,
etc.) as determined by the product of the proportions of affected cases and
controls who have or do not have a particular risk factor.

Reliability   term used to address the internal consistency of a scale item (in
multidimensional scales) and the reproducibility of the scores when the scale
is applied by the same (intra-) or different rater (inter-rater), or by the same
patient (test–retest) in the case of self-rating instruments.[709] The most appropriate method of estimating reliability of a measurement is the test–retest
reproducibility method that examines the agreement between paired ratings
of patients and attributes measured variance to random error.

Remission   definite improvement of signs, symptoms or both, that have been
present for at least 24 hours (e.g. after a relapse). A remission may be complete or incomplete and must last at least one month to be considered

significant for research in therapeutic trials.[191] Remission must be distinguished from transient fluctuations lasting less than 24 hours and from the resolution of paroxysmal symptoms. The onset of a remission may instil a false sense of security in both physician and patient because permanent subtle clinical or subclinical sequelae can commonly be demonstrated postrelapse, and inflammatory disease activity and atrophy may continue despite clinical improvement.

Remyelination   process of repair of damaged myelin. This can be a prominent feature in acute lesions early in the disease course,[422,635,710,711] but becomes less obvious as the disease progresses and recurrent damage occurs. The extent of remyelination in lesions appears to be determined by two factors: the availability of oligoglial progenitor cells and the degree of axonal damage.[517] Lack of remyelination in chronic lesions may be explained by repeated demyelination in the same lesion and exhaustion of the progenitor cell fraction.[179] The speed and effectiveness of remyelination decrease with increasing numbers of demyelinating episodes, and this impairment of remyelination correlates well with a decrease of oligoglial or progenitor cells within the lesions.[712] Intravenous immunoglobulins may promote remyelination within demyelinative lesions induced by Theiler's virus.[713]

Repetition time (TR)   MRI term for the time period between the beginning of one pulse sequence and the beginning of the succeeding and essentially identical pulse sequence at a specified tissue location.

Responsiveness   term used to assess the ability of a scale (e.g. clinical rating scale) to detect meaningful clinical change, preferably over a relatively short period of time.[709] This is done by paired *t*-tests or by measuring effect size [see also *Effect size*].

Retrobulbar neuritis (RBN)   optic neuritis in which the inflammatory plaque is in the part of the optic nerve behind the globe. This is the usual situation in 70–80% of episodes of optic neuritis. The fundal appearances are therefore usually within normal limits [see also *Optic neuritis* and *Optic papillopathy*].

Riluzole   glutamate antagonist with neuroprotective properties that has been shown to delay disease progression in patients with motor neuron disease. In an exploratory cross-over trial in PP MS riluzole seemed to reduce the rate of cervical cord atrophy and the development of hypointense T_1 brain lesions on MRI.[714]

131

Risk factors factors that are known to influence the expected frequency of disease. In MS these include race, HLA type, latitude, familial incidence and age at immigration (e.g. from a low- to high-prevalence region) [see also *Latitude, effects on prevalence, HLA class II, Genetics, influence of* and *Migration*]. The term is also used for those factors (e.g. MRI lesions, oligoclonal bands, abnormal evoked potentials, HLA-DR2 presence) that increase the risk of patients with clinically isolated syndromes progressing to CD MS.

Roquinimex (linomide, quinoline-3-carboxamide) synthetic immuno-modulator that increases the natural killer cell activity associated with increased IFN production.[715] Linomide has been shown to inhibit progression of the disease and to prevent new lesions on MRI.[716,717] Beneficial effects may result from induction of anti-inflammatory cytokines.[718] Phase III trials in the USA and in Europe and Australia were stopped because of unexpected serious cardiovascular events.[719]

Run-in period observation phase (usually 2–6 months) without active treatment, performed before the start of a trial to provide a better estimate of baseline activity, or rarely, to select patients with active disease. Potential advantages include allowing the participants time to become comfortable with personnel and measurement techniques and the identification and minimization of practice effects. Although highly desirable, the extra expense and time involved are considerable disincentives.

S

S-100 beta protein (S100β) nonmyelin protein present in astrocytes and Schwann cells of the central and peripheral nervous system. Elevated plasma levels of S100β are found in MS patients after acute exacerbations.[720] S100β could be a target antigen in MS patients with periphlebitis retinae and uveitis.[721]

Saltatory conduction conduction jumps from one node of Ranvier to the next in normal myelinated fibres and allows signal transmission velocities up to 10 times faster than by continuous conduction in a nerve of equivalent size. The energy requirements in nervous tissue are thus reduced, allowing the transmission of fast trains of impulses.[722]

Sarcoidosis inflammatory disorder of unknown aetiology, commonly affecting young adults and characterized by multiple pulmonary granulomata. Neurological manifestations occur in 5% of patients[723] and include cranial neuropathies, aseptic meningitis, hydrocephalus, hypothalamic dysfunction, intracranial and intraspinal mass lesions, diffuse encephalopathy, vasculopathy, seizures, peripheral neuropathy and myopathy.[723] Spinal cord and optic nerve involvement may be difficult to distinguish from MS. CSF (mild lymphocytosis, normal to elevated protein, elevated IgG index and oligoclonal bands) and MRI abnormalities (periventricular and multifocal white matter lesions) may be indistinguishable.[724] Meningeal involvement, hydrocephalus, hypothalamic or enhancing mass lesions implicate sarcoidosis. A positive chest radiograph, hypercalcaemia, hyperglobulinaemia or anergy on skin testing may support the diagnosis, and diffuse pulmonary uptake on gallium scanning, plus elevated angiotensin converting enzyme (ACE), yields a diagnostic specificity of 83% to 99%.[725]

Schilder's disease (myelinoclastic diffuse sclerosis) rare CNS demyelinating disorder affecting mainly children and usually presenting as an intracranial mass lesion.[726,727] There are at least two subsets of Schilder's disease, the first being a self-limiting monophasic type usually occurring in early adult life and the second a progressive type primarily seen in children that usually culminates in death. Temporary remissions or, very rarely, permanent recovery may occur.[730,731] Some authors believe that Schilder's disease is a distinct and rare form of MS,[729,732] whereas others see it as a separate disorder with the same histopathology as MS. In the absence of a biological marker, the distinction between Schilder's disease, ADEM and MS remains difficult. Clinical history, evidence of viral infection, lesion load, absence or presence of oligoclonal bands and whether the disease is monophasic, progressive, relapsing or remitting, or associated with neuroradiological findings, are all important factors in establishing a definitive diagnosis. The acute lesions of Schilder's disease are similar to those observed in the Marburg variant, but may appear more spongy with cavities or multiple cysts.[290] Neuroimaging studies may demonstrate large, confluent areas of myelin loss often involving an entire lobe or hemisphere and extending to the opposite hemisphere across the corpus callosum.[290] In an attempt to restrict the use of the eponym to diseases identical to the original description by Schilder in 1912,[728] Poser established diagnostic criteria for 'true' Schilder's disease.[729]

Schilder's variant of childhood MS   subset of remitting/relapsing Schilder's disease in which there is also involvement of the spinal cord.[727] [See also *Schilder's disease.*]

Schumacher's criteria   see *Diagnostic criteria, clinical (Schumacher).*

Scripps Neurologic Rating Scale (SNRS)   a 22-item ordinal impairment scale that converts the neurological examination into a numerical score using a three-level scoring system, with scores ranging between 100 (normal) and 0 (worst).[307] This scale is reported to have near normal distribution and a modest responsiveness to clinical change.[186,733] Some studies have suggested skewed distribution, high rater variability and low responsiveness, but high correlation with the EDSS, the functional Independence Measure and the Cambridge Basic Multiple Sclerosis Score.[32] [See *Appendix 2.*]

Secondary progressive MS (SP MS)   disease course characterized by progression (with or without occasional superimposed relapses, minor remissions or plateaux) after an initial relapsing–remitting disease course.[127] Progression (i.e. steadily worsening disability) must not be relapse-related and must occur between relapses in patients with superimposed attacks. The distinction from a step-wise, relapse-related deterioration can be difficult particularly in the later stages of RR MS when neurological deficits may accumulate and merge after relapses. Approximately 50% of RR MS patients will enter the phase of SP MS within 10 years and 80% within 20 years of disease onset.

Self-tolerance   the lack of immune responsiveness to self-antigens. Its breakdown is a feature of auto-immune disease.

Sensory symptoms   most patients experience sensory loss or alteration at some time. Symptoms include dysaesthesiae, paraesthesiae, numbness, pain and various distortions of sensation. Tactile perception may be reduced as though there is something between stimulus and skin ('like a film or glove'). Tight swollen sensations around limbs or trunk are caused by lesions in the posterior columns of the spinal cord. Unpleasant sensory distortions (dysaesthesiae), including burning, stinging, sensations of wetness or insect-like movement sensations under the skin (formication) are due to lesions in the spinothalamic tracts. Tingling ('pins and needles') paraesthesiae may occur from lesions in the lateral or posterior columns of the spinal cord. [See also *Dysaesthetic extremity pain*.]

Sex   see *Gender*.

Sexual dysfunction   is a common finding in MS and reported to be one of the most distressing aspects of disability in up to 91% of men and 72% of women.[286] Many patients experience orgasmic difficulties due to transient or permanent erectile dysfunction or decreased libido.[286,737,738] Contributing factors are multiple and complex and include the location of lesions in the CNS, sensory loss, disability, spasticity, pain, fatigue and psychosocial and endocrine factors.[738] The frequency of sexual dysfunction is reported to be correlated with pyramidal tract symptoms and bladder disturbances.[737,739]

Shadow plaque   area in the white matter characterized by the presence of thin myelin sheaths which usually stains paler with a myelin stain than the surrounding normal white matter.[740] They may take the form of a hazy rim or crescent adjacent to the margin of a more defined chronic plaque. These areas are considered to be incompletely demyelinated or areas of remyelination.[11]

Short inversion-time inversion-recovery sequence (STIR) MRI technique that produces images in which T_1- and T_2-dependent contrasts are additive. STIR imaging is used to suppress the signal of fat, reducing chemical shift artefacts caused by high-signal-intensity subcutaneous adipose tissue.[741] With this sequence used in combination with coronal imaging, it has been possible to detect optic nerve lesions in the majority of patients with optic neuritis.[741,742]

Short-term (immediate) memory digit span has been found to be mildly impaired in some studies of MS patients[447,448] and normal in others.[210,234] The registration and storage of information in immediate memory may be reasonably intact unless patients are in relapse or severely disabled.[449] [See also *Working memory*.]

Silent MS patients with no known symptoms appropriate to MS during life in whom the diagnosis of MS is made by chance at autopsy,[182] or, coincidentally, by neuroimaging.

Single nucleotide polymorphism (SNP) once in every few hundred base pairs there is a biallelic polymorphism in the sequence caused by a single base-pair change. These polymorphisms occur in both coding and noncoding regions and usefully, perhaps once in 1000 base pairs. These usually account for neutral substitutions that can be identified and used to specify haplotypes carrying specific susceptibility alleles.

Sjögren's syndrome common rheumatological disorder characterized by the presence of xerostomia and keratoconjunctivitis with or without other evidence of connective tissue disorder. Some patients with CNS involvement may have clinical, CSF, evoked potential and MRI abnormalities that can closely resemble MS.[743,744] However, the peak incidence occurs in the fifth to sixth decades and cranial neuropathies and neuromuscular features are common. Rheumatoid factor, antinuclear antibodies and anti-Ro antibodies may be present; Ro/SS-A and La/SS-B antibodies are specific findings in Sjögren's syndrome.[745]

Sodium channels negatively charged and specifically selective channels for the passage of sodium ions that are essential mediators of both depolarization and repolarization of the nerve membrane during an action potential. They are concentrated at the node of Ranvier with a density of up to 50

136

times that of the internodal membrane. The re-establishment of sodium channels in the axon membrane is one of the mechanisms that may restore nonsaltatory conduction and improve function in demyelinated lesions.

Somatosensory evoked potential (SEP) electrical responses in the brain and spinal cord elicited by electrical shocks applied to a peripheral nerve, most commonly the median or tibial nerve. The pathways subserving SEP include the posterior columns, medial lemnisci and internal capsules.[746] Peak latency and amplitude abnormalities can help determine the anatomical level of disturbance along these sensory pathways. *Table 17* summarizes the frequency of abnormality for median and tibial nerve SEP in MS patients. SEP may be normal in patients with solely positive sensory symptoms, e.g. paraesthesiae,[215] or impaired vibration sense.[360] Patients with suspected MS with abnormal SEP are 2.4 to 3.9 times as likely to develop CD MS as patients with normal SEP.[586,747]

Space–time cluster analysis epidemiological model used as a general test of a possible infectious aetiology based on time and place of residence at the onset of disease.[200] For diseases with a long latency such as MS, it is based on a particular age, or at some time preceding disease onset (i.e. related to a possible susceptibility period). Only two of six published studies have found significant clustering, at 21 to 23 years of age[345] and 13 to 20 years,[748] which might suggest an infectious or toxic factor in the aetiology of MS.

Spasticity velocity-dependent increase in the tonic stretch reflex which forms one component of the upper motor neurone syndrome.[749] Increased muscle tone particularly affects the extensor muscles of the upper limbs and the flexor muscles of the lower limbs. Spasticity occurs frequently in MS, impairing mobility and causing muscle spasms, with or without pain, and disturbed sleep. Patients usually refer to problems with limb stiffness and clumsiness [see also *Baclofen* and *Tizanidine*].

SPECTRIMS (Rebif®, Serono International SA) phase III trial of INFβ-1a involving 618 patients with SP MS who received subcutaneous injection of two doses (22 and 44 μg) three times weekly for three years.[750] Annual relapse rate was significantly reduced in patients with treatment (0.71 vs 0.50, $P < 0.001$), but treatment with IFNβ-1a did not significantly affect disability progression in this study. The reduction in relapse rate was associated with a significant reduction in numbers of active lesions, combined unique

137

activity and the accumulation of burden of disease (BOD) on MRI.[751] The lack of efficacy on disability despite dramatic effects on relapses supports the notion that clinical disability results from axonal damage, which may become independent of inflammation as MS progresses.[89,181] Thus, anti-inflammatory treatment early in the disease course (i.e. RR), when relapses are usually more frequent, is likely to be more effective at preventing disability than in the latter stages of the disease [see also *ETOMS* and *PRISMS*].

Speech disturbances   see *Dysarthria*.

Spin density   one of the principal determinants of the strength of the MR signal, i.e. the higher the spin density, the higher the signal intensity. The MR observable proton density shows a complex relationship to hydrogen or water concentration.

Spin echo imaging (spin echo sequence, conventional spin echo)   magnetic resonance imaging of a spin echo formed by a sequence of radiofrequency pulses consisting of a 90° excitation pulse followed by a 180° echo rephasing pulse. One echo is usually used for T_1-weighting using shorter repetition times, TR [see *Repetition time*], while two echoes are used to generate proton density [see *Spin density*] with shorter echo times, TE [see *Echo time*] and T_2-weighting [see *T_2-weighted imaging*] with longer TE and longer TR. The characteristics of MS lesions are best demonstrated by proton density or T_2-weighted images. T_2-weighted images are the most commonly used for diagnosis (see *MRI diagnostic criteria*) and secondary outcomes in clinical trials (either T_2 activity, i.e. new or enlarging T_2 lesions, or total lesion load known as burden of disease).[3]

Spinal cord compression   benign tumours, including neurofibroma and meningioma, or degenerative spine disease, may mimic acute or chronic spinal MS. Loss of reflexes, radicular pain, segmental sensory loss and segmental muscle wasting are alerting signs. A progressive paraparesis with or without these features and without evidence of dissemination in space and time requires exclusion of a compressive cause, generally by spinal MRI.

Spinocerebellar degeneration   see *Hereditary spinocerebellar ataxia*.

Steroids   see *Corticosteroids or glucocorticosteroids*.

Stress proteins   variety of polypeptides synthesized by cells in response to injury. In MS, these proteins can be recognized by specific T-cell-mediated autoimmune reactions and augment inflammation and tissue damage in MS.[752] Certain stress proteins, such as heat shock protein-65 and α-B-crystallin are highly enriched in oligodendrocytes in MS lesions.[752,753] Other stress proteins including heat shock protein-27 and -70[754] or c-fos[755] are mainly present in astrocytes and inflammatory cells.

Subacute combined degeneration of the spinal cord   a system degeneration caused by deficiency of vitamin B_{12}, which involves both the lateral and posterior columns of the spinal cord. Features of a peripheral neuropathy usually precede the signs of CNS involvement. Presentation is with ascending paraesthesiae, instability of gait, impaired joint position and vibration sense, followed by a symmetric paraparesis with, usually, decreased tendon reflexes and extensor plantar responses. Vitamin B_{12} absorption is reduced (antibodies to intrinsic factor may be present) and serum levels are low. Disturbed vitamin B_{12} metabolism and low serum levels of B_{12} have been reported.[756] Rarely, a similar syndrome may be caused by folic acid deficiency.

Subacute myelo-optic neuritis (SMON)   disease attributed to chronic clioquinol treatment for gastro-intestinal disturbance, usually in travellers and mostly confined to Japanese.[757]

Subcortical dementia   dementia characterized by slow information processing, impaired memory retrieval, deficient problem solving and personality and mood disturbances, rather than the aphasia, apraxia and agnosia found in a cortical dementia such as Alzheimer's disease.[758] Rao suggested that the pattern of cognitive impairment in MS is similar to that seen in Huntington's disease, Parkinson's disease and progressive supranuclear palsy.[759] Disruption of the white-matter connections between the frontal lobes and subcortical structures may be responsible for the shared cognitive and emotional characteristics of the subcortical dementias.[760] [See also *Cognitive dysfunction*.]

Suicide   appears to be increased in MS, but rates are probably under-reported. A 7.5-fold increase in suicide compared with a matched population was reported from Canadian clinics[761] and double the expected rates in another population-based Danish study.[762] [See also *Depression*.]

Sulfasalazine nonsteroidal anti-inflammatory and immunomodulatory drug that is effective in several inflammatory diseases.[763] Sulfasalazine did not prevent disease progression in a randomized, double-blind, placebo-controlled phase III trial of 199 patients with active relapsing–remitting or progressive MS.[764] Interestingly, a two-year interim analysis in this study demonstrated a temporary improvement in relapse-related outcomes, without providing sustained slowing of EDSS progression at three years. This indicates that MS trials should be of sufficient length to determine a meaningful impact on disease course.

Survival number of patients in a specific cohort who have not yet reached a defined endpoint. It is dependend on full ascertainment of incidence and prevalence cases.

Susac's syndrome very rare small-vessel vasculitis affecting young females and characterized by a steroid-responsive stupor or coma, retinal ischaemic lesions, deafness, MRI lesions in white matter and livido reticularis. Permanent deafness and cognitive sequelae can be severe. It is a self-limiting disease that may relapse and remit and is often misdiagnosed as MS.

Suspected MS diagnostic category in the McDonald and Halliday classification [see also *Diagnostic criteria, clinical*].

Syphilis venereal disease caused by infection with the spirochaete *Treponema pallidum*. Meningovascular syphilis is characterized by a relapsing illness with stroke and characteristic capsular lesions involving the adjacent basal ganglia on MRI. Tabes dorsalis is now rare due to early treatment of syphilis and is characterized by ataxia, spasticity and dementia with small, unreactive pupils. Cellular reaction with high protein in the CSF is an important indicator of active disease and diagnosis is confirmed by the demonstration of intrathecal production of *T. pallidum*-specific IgG antibodies.[765]

Systemic lupus erythematosus (SLE) commonest connective tissue disorder mimicking MS, characterized by antibodies against components of cell nuclei. It is a multisystem disease causing arthralgia, rashes, CNS and renal disease. MS may be mimicked when neurological involvement is dominant and fever, weight loss and involvement of skin, joint and kidney are absent. Multifocal CNS lesions, particularly optic neuritis and myelopathy and/or a relapsing–remitting disease course, may be confusing. Neuropsychiatric features occurring in SLE that are uncommon in MS, particularly as present-ing symptoms, include dementia, psychosis, affective disorders and encephalopathy. Oligoclonal bands have been found in 42% of cases with SLE[766] and cranial MRI may not be distinguishable from MS,[767] although the lesions in SLE usually predominate in subcortical white matter.[291] Serological tests for SLE are not distinctive and antinuclear factor has been found in approximately 30% of patients with MS.[768] Antiribosomal P protein anti-bodies with CNS involvement in SLE, especially those with lupus psychosis, are highly specific to SLE.[769]

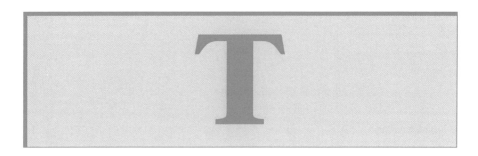

Tap 1 and 2 genes   peptide transporter genes encoded at the centromeric end of class II HLA. An association between Tap 1 and 2 genes and MS has not been demonstrated.[770,771]

T-cell receptor (TCR)   specific glycoprotein receptor on the cell surface of T cells that allows recognition of antigens. The TCR is composed of either an α- and a β-chain, or a γ- and a δ-chain. Thus T cells may be either αβ T cells or γδ T cells, depending on their receptor type. T cells expressing the αβ T-cell receptor constitute >95% of the T cells in blood, while the γδ receptor is a far less common receptor. Both classes of T cell are consistently found in inflammatory infiltrates in MS.[772] [See *Figure 20.*]

T-cell receptor gene (TCR gene)   highly variable glycoproteins encoded on different loci of chromosome [see also *T-cell receptor*]. As with genetic organization of immunoglobulin, the T-cell receptor has variable (V), joining (J) and constant (C) regions and diversity (D) segments. The β-chain gene complex is encoded on chromosome 7q32, the α-chain locus on chromosome 14q11 and the δ-chain gene between the V and J regions of a chain. The γ chain gene maps to chromosome 7q32. There is insufficient evidence to confirm whether a susceptibility gene for MS is encoded within the T-cell receptor α[773-775] or β[776,777] loci.

T cells   see *T lymphocytes*.

T-cell vaccination   a therapeutic strategy designed to induce an immune response against T cells (or T-cell receptor protein) supposedly involved in causing MS. Several exploratory trials have been reported with mixed results. Larger phase II studies are required.[840]

T cytotoxic cells (Tc)   T lymphocytes that are usually CD8+ and recognize antigens through the T cell receptor in an MHC class I restricted fashion,

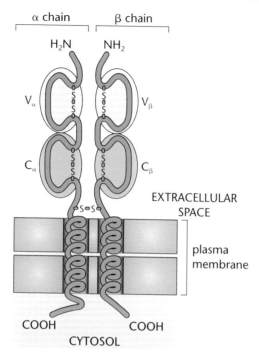

Figure 20 **T-cell receptor:** A T-cell receptor heterodymer. Reproduced with permission.[21A]

usually on cells that have become neoplastic or infected by viruses [see *T lymphocytes*].

T-helper cells (Th) see *T lymphocytes*.

T-helper 0 cells (Th0) subset of CD4$^+$ cells in both humans and mice based on cytokine production and effector functions. Th0 cells synthesize multiple cytokines with an intermediate (mixed) pattern between those of Th1 and Th2 cells. The term may be used in reference to undifferentiated precursors of Th1 or Th2 cells (preferably denoted as Thn, indicating neutral).

T-helper 1 cells (Th1) subset of CD4$^+$ cells that synthesize IL-2, IFN-γ and TNF-α, or especially TNF-β (lymphotoxin-α) that are involved in cell-mediated immunity.[167] Th1 and Th2 responses are usually reciprocally inhibitory.[167] The major inducer of Th1 responses is interleukin-12 (IL-12). EAE is mediated by Th1 cells so that blocking Th1 development (e.g. by IL-12 suppression) prevents EAE.[614,778] Likewise, MS is believed to be dependent on an activation of Th1 cells that is not sufficiently counterbalanced by

Th2 cells.[779,780] Enhanced Th1 responses have been shown in MS, although there are still some discrepancies within the Th1/Th2 model.[781]

T-helper 2 cells (Th2)   subset of CD4⁺ T cells that synthesize IL-4, IL-5, IL-6, IL-9, IL-10 and IL-13 and exert their primary function in humoral immune reactions[167,782] [see also *CD4⁺ T cells* and *T-helper 1 cells*]. Th2 cytokines generally inhibit Th1 responses. Administration of Th2 cytokine IL-4 suppresses EAE. Moreover, endogenous Th2 cytokines may be important for the resistance to Th1-mediated autoimmune diseases such as EAE.[783]

T-helper 3 cells (Th3)   subtype of immunoregulatory T-helper cells similar to Th2 cells but producing, in addition, high amounts of the cytokine TGF-β.[784]

T lymphocytes (T cells)   thymus-derived lymphocytes that confer cell-mediated immunity. They co-operate with B lymphocytes, enabling them to synthesize antibodies. T cells are subdivided according to their expression of CD4 or CD8 surface molecules [see *Figure 21*]. CD4 cells recognize antigen in association with class II MHC molecules and largely function as T-helper (Th) cells.[163] CD8 cells recognize antigen in association with class I MHC molecules and largely function as T-cytotoxic (Tc) cells.[163] After a Th cell recognizes and interacts with an antigen-MHC II molecule complex on the membrane of the antigen-presenting cell, the cell is activated and secretes various cytokines, which, in turn, activate B cells, Tc cells, macrophages and various other cells that participate in the immune response [see also *CD4*, *CD8*, *Major histocompatibility complex*, *Antigen-presenting cell* and *Cytokines*].

T_1-lesion load   estimated volume or area of gadolinium enhanced lesions on T_1-weighted imaging [see *Gadolinium-enhancing lesion*].

T_1-relaxation time, MRI   longitudinal magnetization recovers to its equilibrium (steady-state) value with time constant T_1 resulting from the interaction of a spinning nucleus with its physical surroundings or lattice (hence also called spin–lattice relaxation). Marked prolongation of T_1 relaxation time has been reported in MS lesions[785] and normal-appearing white matter,[628,786] and correlated with enlargement of the extracellular space, which occurs as a result of axonal loss or oedema.[878]

T_1-weighted imaging   MR sequence such as short TR/short TE spin-echo or inversion recovery designed to distinguish tissues with different T_1-relaxation times [see also *Black holes* and *Gadolinium-enhancing lesion*].

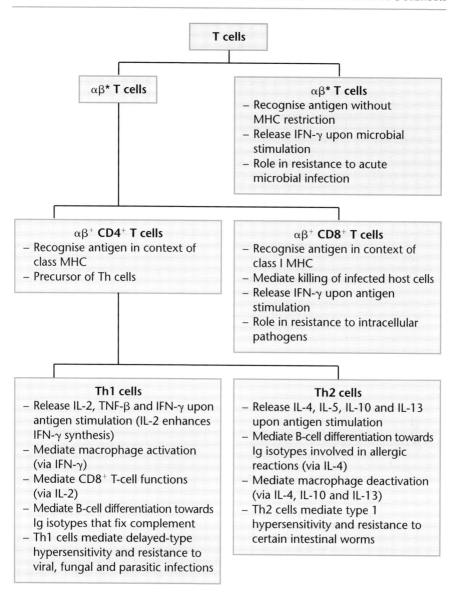

Figure 21 **T lymphocytes:** Overview of the different types of T cells. T cells expressing the αβ T-cell receptor (αβ⁺ T cells) constitute >95% of the T cells in blood. The rare γδ⁺ T cells are slightly enriched in certain multiple sclerosis lesions (e.g. Selmaj et al.[536]). The αβ⁺ T cells can be subdivided into CD4⁺ and CD8⁺ cells, and the CD4⁺ T cells can be divided into Th1 and Th2 cells. Reproduced with permission.[21]

T$_2$ active lesion   new, recurrent, newly enlarging, or persistently enlarging lesions detected on serial PD/T$_2$ scans.[334] Reductions of 67% (22 μg) and 78% (44 μg) in the median number of T$_2$ active lesions are observed in MS patients treated with INFβ-1a (Rebif®).[213]

T$_2$ decay curve analysis   multi-exponential MRI analysis that converts decay curves into distributions of T$_2$ components using statistical methodology. By using this sequence it is possible to obtain multiple points on the T$_2$ decay curve from approximately 10 ms out to seconds and the data are then analysed via fitting to several exponential curves.[785] This method may help to increase the specificity of the evaluation of high intensity abnormalities in MS.[567] Earlier studies of the T$_2$ decay curve of normal white matter indicate a best-fit to a monoexponential curve, whereas that of visible lesions best fits a biexponential T$_2$ relaxation time, reflecting myelin loss with enlargement of the extracellular space and gliosis.[785,787,788] Prolongation of T$_2$ relaxation time in the normal appearing white matter has been reported in MS[628,789] [see also *T$_2$ relaxation time* and *Magnetic resonance imaging*]. Previously the literature contained many conflicting and confusing results, mostly due to the use of inappropriate measurement and analysis techniques. Using a 32-echo technique, MacKay et al.[790] distinguished three water reservoirs in normal white matter: (a) a small component with a short T$_2$ between 10 and 50 ms due to water compartmentalized in myelin membranes, so-called myelin water; (b) a major component with T$_2$ between 70 ms and 95 ms due to water in cytoplasmic and extracellular spaces; (c) CSF with T$_2$ of 1 s or more. Myelin water depicted by the short T$_2$ component of the T$_2$-relaxation distribution can be displayed as a map of brain myelin. Such myelin water maps have been shown to correspond to the expected anatomical distribution of myelin in normal volunteers. MS lesions in patients have shown varying levels of this short T$_2$ component, ranging from normal to reduced or absent.

T$_2$ relaxation time   transverse magnetization decays with time constant T$_2$ resulting from the interactions of the spinning nuclei with the spin of identical nuclei pointing in the opposite direction (hence also called spin–spin relaxation) with loss of coherence. Significantly increased T$_2$ relaxation time has been reported in MRI studies of MS lesions[785] and normal-appearing white matter.[628,788,789]

T$_2$-weighted imaging   MR sequence such as a spin echo with a long TR/long TE designed to distinguish tissues with different T$_2$ relaxation times. T$_2$-weighted

146

images are the most frequently used routine diagnostic MRI technique [see also *MRI diagnostic criteria*] and have applications for prognosis[199] and secondary outcomes in clinical trials [see *Total lesion load* and *Burden of disease*].

T₂-weighted lesion load   see *Total lesion load*.

T4 antigen   old terminology for CD4 [see also *CD4*].

T8 antigen   old terminology for CD8 [see also *CD8*].

Three-tier composite   see *MS functional composite*.

Timed 25-Foot Walk (T25W)   quantitative measure of lower limb function and ambulation, in which the patient is asked to walk a clearly marked 25-foot course. The time taken to complete the course is recorded.[572] It has been considered a precise and sensitive measure of ambulatory impairment in MS[572] and is one component of the MSFC,[573] but there may be problems with test–retest reliability.[792] [See *Appendix 4*.]

Tizanidine (Zanaflex) α_2-noradrenergic agonist that has been shown to have antispasticity effects in double-blind trials.[793–795] It has similar efficacy to baclofen when given at a 1 : 2 ratio (mg tizanidine : mg baclofen), but may cause less apparent limb weakness.[796]

TNF gene   see *Tumour necrosis factor gene*.

Tolerance   antigen-specific unresponsiveness of T or B cells. It can be central vs peripheral and can be achieved via diverse mechanisms, including clonal deletion, anergy, active suppression and receptor editing.

Tonic spasm (tonic seizure)   common paroxysmal symptom in MS that begins as a muscle spasm in the limbs or trunk and spreads upward or downwards, at times crossing the midline. The spasm may be preceded by an intense pain or unpleasant burning or tingling sensation, starting abruptly in the involved extremity or trunk. During an attack, the fingers and elbow are flexed and the lower limb (if involved) is extended at all joints. Pain in the affected limbs may be frequent and severe.[797] Ephaptic activation of fibres in the lateral corticospinal tracts may be responsible.[660] [See also *Paroxysmal syndromes*.]

Total lesion load (TLL)   total area or volume of abnormal hyperintense lesions measured from conventional proton density/T₂-weighted images [see

147

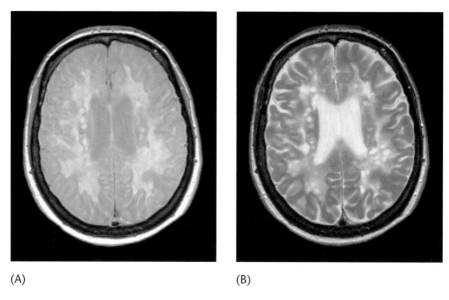

(A)   (B)

Figure 22 **Total lesion load:** A: Proton-density; B: T$_2$-weighted images in clinically definite multiple sclerosis showing areas of confluent abnormality as well as discrete lesions.

also *Spin density* and *T$_2$-weighted imaging*] [see *Figure 22*], also known as the burden of disease (BOD). TLL measurements may be used as a secondary endpoint to monitor treatment efficacy in large-scale phase III clinical trials in MS.[3] TLL has little pathological specificity and can represent oedema, inflammation, gliosis, demyelination or tissue and axonal loss.[567] Most serial studies show only weak to modest correlation between changes in TLL and clinical disability.[139] TLL provides prognostic value in predicting subsequent disease activity and levels of disability.[126,199,798]

Toxicity trials   see *Phase I treatment trial.*

Transforming growth factor beta (TGF-β)   polypeptide produced by transformed cells, activated T lymphocytes, B cells, and macrophages that has suppressive effects on both T- and B-cell-related immunity.[488] Its potent immunosuppressive properties include downregulation of IFNγ-induced class II MHC expression, inhibition cytotoxicity and, possibly, inhibition of TNF.[799] Impaired production of TGF-β has been associated with disease activity.[800,801] Stimulating the production of TGF-β might be one of the mechanisms by which IFN-β mediates its positive treatment effects.[802,803] However, a phase I/II trial of TGF-β treatment in 11 patients with MS showed no clinical or MRI effects.[804]

Transverse myelitis   acute, severe, inflammatory, demyelinating lesion of the spinal cord, characterized by a rapidly evolving paraparesis (often to complete paraplegia), a sensory level on the trunk and retention of urine. One-third of patients report a preceding infectious illness or vaccination. Spinal involvement is usually bilateral, severe and symmetric, whereas acute spinal cord lesions due to MS are usually partial and asymmetric.[805] On long-term follow-up only a minority of patients with transverse myelitis eventually develop MS.[805] By contrast, most of those with incomplete cord syndromes (typically quasi Brown–Séquard syndromes) develop MS.[126]

Treatment failure   outcome measure based on a defined level of worsening which, once reached, deems the treatment to be regarded as unsuccessful. It is generally included in a therapeutic trial to allow patients to discontinue the study and receive an alternative, hopefully more effective, treatment. In MS trials it has often been based on the outcome measure confirmed progression. Thus the probability of a confirmed worsening of 1 point for patients with baseline EDSS < 5.5, and of 0.5 point for patients with baseline EDSS ≥ 5.5 and ≤ 7.0 has been considered as a significant clinical deterioration and a criterion for treatment failure.[224] This definition is based on observations that staying times at EDSS 6 and 7 are substantially longer than at EDSS 3, 4, and 5.[806] Unfortunately, confirmed progression is not a hard endpoint as a proportion of patients who become treatment failures subsequently remit.[225]

Trends analysis   a categorical method of analysing outcome of therapeutic trials that compares treatment effects within statistically separable subgroups defined according to the direction of their in-trial disability change.[225] The advantages are that all the serial disability data acquired in a trial are utilized (thus taking into account *all* the disability changes) and a 'numbers-needed-to-treat' analysis is possible [see also *Numbers needed to treat*]. The method requires validation over longer periods. Other disease course analysis models have also been described.[370,807,808]

Trigeminal neuralgia   episodic, severe unilateral facial pain in MS, occurring in bouts usually lasting less than 5 minutes, but recurring several times a day. Pain is spontaneous or triggered by wind, touch, chewing or talking. It is characteristically stabbing, electric shock-like or lancinating. It has been attributed to inflammatory lesions involving the trigeminal nucleus or root entry zone.[809] Pathophysiological mechanisms include ephaptic spread secondary to demyelination[660] and release of inflammatory cytokines by cells within MS plaques.[554] Coincidental pathologies such as tumours and 'vascular compression' may also cause similar neuralgic facial pain in MS and require exclusion. Conventional medical treatment includes carbamazepine, phenytoin and gabapentin. Some patients require surgical or electrolytic lesions. [See also *Paroxysmal syndromes*.]

Trimolecular complex combination of antigen, T cell receptor and major histocompatibility complex,[810] that is required to activate T cells. Antigens recognized by T cells must have two distinct interaction sites: one, the epitope, interacts with the T-cell receptor and the other, called the agretope, interacts with an MHC molecule [see *Figure 23*].

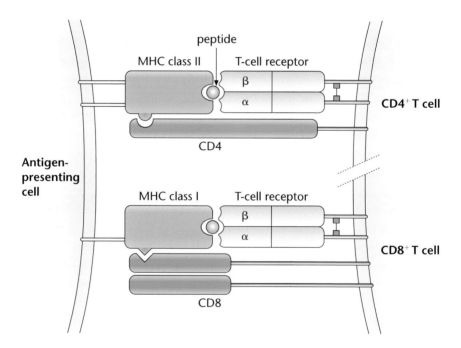

Figure 23 **Trimolecular complex**: Antigen recognition by CD4⁺ T cells and CD8⁺ T cells. The T-cell receptor of CD4⁺ T cells recognizes an antigen peptide to an MHC class II molecule (e.g. HLA-DR, -DP or -DQ) on the surface of an antigen-presenting cell. The T cell receptor of CD8⁺ T cells recognizes an antigen peptide bound to an MHC class I molecule (e.g. HLA-A, -B or -C). CD4 and CD8 act as coreceptors. Reproduced with permission.[21]

Troiano Scale 'functional scale' used in one therapeutic MS trial[315] which is heavily weighted for ambulation and does not assess visual, cognitive, affective, bladder and bowel disabilities. No reliability and validity data are available.

Tropical spastic paraparesis see *HTLV-I associated myelopathy*.

Tryptizol see *Amitriptyline*.

Tumour necrosis factor alpha (TNF-α) pro-inflammatory cytokine thought to be involved in the inflammatory response and tissue injury in MS.[811] TNF-α has been demonstrated within active MS lesions,[812] and elevated TNF-α levels in the serum and CSF have been correlated with exacerbations and disease progression.[535,813–815] Furthermore, TNF-α treatment worsens EAE[811] and its neutralization by anti-TNF antibody treatment protects animals.[514,515,816] However, gene targeted mice doubly deficient in TNF-α and the closely related cytokine lymphotoxin-α (TNF-β), which uses the same receptor, retain full susceptibility to EAE.[817] Moreover, the hypothesis that neutralization of TNF-α may reduce or halt MS progression could not be proven in a phase II study of Lenercept (anti-TNF antibody) in MS patients.[516] IFN-β therapy may be associated with a diminished serum level of TNF-α in MS.[818]

Tumour necrosis factor beta (TNF-β) see *Lymphotoxin*.

Tumour necrosis factor gene (TNF gene) gene located near the HLA class III region, between HLA class I and class II genes on chromosome 6. Evidence suggests that TNF is involved in the pathogenesis of MS,[493,535,814,815] but genetic variants of TNF have not been associated with MS susceptibility.[819–821] [See also *Lymphotoxin* and *Tumour necrosis factor alpha*.]

Turbo gradient spin echo (TGSE) very fast MRI sequence that can acquire brain images in less than one minute. May be useful for scanning claustrophobic and uncooperative patients for diagnostic purposes, but has low sensitivity and poor reproducibility.[382,822]

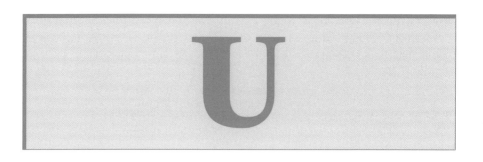

U-fibres   short myelinated arcuate fibres that either connect axons in adjacent or nearby areas of cortex, or on one side of a sulcus or gyrus to the other. They are commonly involved in MS by lesions that occur near the cortico-medullary boundary between white and grey matter [see also *Juxtacortical lesion*].

Uhthoff's symptom   transient blurring of vision with loss of colour saturation associated with exertion or body temperature change (e.g. hot bath), characteristic of a demyelinating optic nerve lesion. Symptoms usually occur within 5 to 20 minutes of exposure to the provoking factor and resolve within 5 to 60 minutes of resting or cooling. Reductions of the VEP amplitude of 68% have been shown to coincide with the Uhthoff's phenomenon.[824] The underlying mechanism is thought to be a temperature-dependent conduction block occurring in demyelinated, and thus poorly insulated, fibres. The incidence in the course of ON may be 50%,[646] but it may also occur in the absence of previous or concurrent ON. Uhthoff's symptom may indicate a poor prognosis for recurrent attacks of ON and the early development of MS.[646] Other visual or nonvisual symptoms (e.g. paraesthesiae or weakness) are also prone to similar temperature-related, transient worsening.

Unidentified bright objects (UBOs)   descriptive term for areas of increased signal of unknown aetiology on T_2-weighted images.

United Kingdom Neurological Disability Scale (UKNDS)   see *Guy's Neurological Disability Scale*.

Urge incontinence   involuntary passing of urine associated with a sensation of an imminent desire to urinate. [See also *Bladder dysfunction* and *Detrusor hyperreflexia*.]

Urgency of micturition   inability to consciously suppress the sensation of an imminent desire to urinate. In MS the cause is a small, spastic bladder. There is often associated frequency and incontinence ('urge incontinence'). [See also *Bladder dysfunction* and *Detrusor hyperreflexia*.]

Urinary hesitancy   inability or difficulty in the initiation of voluntary voiding. [See also *Bladder dysfunction* and *Detrusor areflexia*.]

Urodynamics   measurement of the functional activities involved in micturition. For example, a cystometrogram combined with a simultaneous assessment of urine flow rate and perineal electromyography can identify many bladder and sphincteric abnormalities. In a meta-analysis of 22 series of 1882 MS patients the incidence of abnormal urodynamic findings was 90%.[286] The three common patterns of urodynamic abnormality in MS are detrusor hyperreflexia, detrusor areflexia and detrusor–sphincter dyssynergia. [See also *Bladder dysfunction, Detrusor areflexia, Detrusor hyperreflexia* and *Detrusor–sphincter dyssynergia*.]

153

V

Validity extent to which an instrument measures the construct it purports to measure.[709] Various types of validity have been defined and discussed in detail.[825,826] There are many methods of gathering evidence for the validity of a measure, but construct validity is used in the absence of a gold standard to assess clinical scales in MS [see also *Construct validity*].

Vascular cell adhesion molecule-1 (VCAM-1) member of the immunoglobulin supergene family that is preferentially involved in T-cell binding to the endothelium.[827] An increased expression of VCAM-1 in MS lesions supports a role in inflammatory lesion development.[534] Accumulating evidence shows increased serum and cerebrospinal fluid levels of soluble VCAM-1 in MS, which correlate with clinical and MRI markers of disease activity.[20,457]

Vascular fibrosis feature of all neurological conditions associated with chronic brain inflammation and present in MS plaques, mostly in long-standing disease.[501] The presence of vascular fibrosis may facilitate the removal of inflammatory cells from chronically inflamed brain lesions in MS.[517]

Vasculitis vascular inflammation may be seen as a primary event in the evolution of the disease of MS. The venular wall is infiltrated with mononuclear cells and perivascular accumulations of leukocytes are associated with leakage of serum proteins, upregulation of adhesion molecules on endothelial cells and some deposition of complement components on the luminal surface of the vessel wall.[517] In some exceptionally inflammatory cases of MS, occlusive and haemorrhagic vascular changes have been described.[828]

Vestibular neuronitis acute disturbance of vestibular function, characterized by a paroxysmal attack or attacks of vertigo with prostration, nausea and vomiting, but without tinnitus, deafness or cranial nerve signs. Absence of caloric reaction may be demonstrated in vestibular neuronitis.

Visual evoked potential (VEP)   series of potentials recorded from the occipital region in response to visual stimuli, most often a checkerboard pattern of black and white squares that reverse at 2 Hz ('pattern-reversal' stimulation). The VEP is approximately twice as sensitive as MRI for detecting abnormalities in the optic nerves, chiasm and optic tract[566,829] and can provide paraclinical evidence of dissemination of subclinical abnormalities in sensory pathways to assist the diagnosis.[191] Abnormal prolongation of the latency of the major positive wave (P100) is present in over 90% of patients with a history of acute optic neuritis[357] and in the majority of patients with CD MS.[148] The frequency of abnormalities decreases from definite to probable to possible cases[148] (*Table* 17). Studies have demonstrated a significant association between abnormal VEP and an increased risk of developing CD MS.[586,747] [See also *P100*.]

Visual field defect   area of reduced or lost vision within the visual field. The classical field defect seen in 76–81% of patients presenting with optic neuritis is a central scotoma.[55,830] This may resolve to a paracentral (relative) desaturation scotoma (i.e. detectable with a red coloured test object). The most commonly observed field defects in the optic neuritis treatment trial were areas of diffuse depression (48%) or localized defects including altitudinal (15%), quadrantic (6%), central and centrocaecal (8%) abnormalities.[56,831,832] Most of the visual field defects in patients with ON recover within 6 months whether they are initially localized or diffuse, mild or severe.[831,832]

Visual linear scale   self-rating method for measuring symptoms (e.g. fatigue) on a visual analogue or visual linear scale. Patients rate symptom severity on a scale of 1 to 10, or by placing a mark somewhere on a line between 'no symptoms' and 'severe symptoms'.[365]

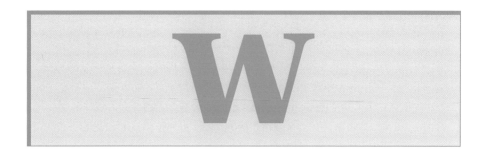

Wallerian degeneration   anterograde degeneration of axons and their myelin sheaths after proximal axonal or cell body injury. Some MS damage, particularly in the spinal cord, may be attributed to Wallerian degeneration.[833]

Washington Committee criteria   see *Diagnostic criteria, clinical (Poser)*.

Wave V   one of five major waves usually identifiable in the BAEP. The loss of amplitude or disappearance of wave V is one of the typical abnormalities found in MS.[834] [See also *Brainstem auditory evoked potential*.]

Whipple's disease   multisystem disorder caused by infection with the bacillus *Tropheryma whippelii*. It is characterized by steatorrhoea, abdominal pain, weight loss, arthritis and lymphadenopathy. The most common CNS features are dementia, seizures and midbrain syndromes, including a characteristic movement disorder, oculo-masticatory myorrhythmia. Most patients respond to antibacterial therapy. This disease can produce MRI appearances indistinguishable from MS (e.g. multifocal white matter lesions), but caudate nucleus and putamen may be involved.[291]

Working memory (WM)   system that provides temporary storage and manipulation of information necessary for such complex tasks as language comprehension, learning and reasoning.[835] WM capacity, as measured by the digit span task and the Brown–Peterson interference task, was reported to be normal or near normal in MS,[449,836,837] but objective event-related potential studies using specific memory paradigms have demonstrated that up to one-third of patients presenting with isolated spinal cord syndromes due to MS already have abnormalities of WM.[355]

Worsening to EDSS 3.0   endpoint measure based on measure of moderate disability. The median time for the total MS population to reach this level of disability is approximately 8 years from diagnosis.[301]

Worsening to EDSS 6.0 relatively firm endpoint based on the requirement for unilateral ambulatory assistance (e.g. stick or cane), an important milestone in disease progression in MS.[301,838] Analysis in placebo groups shows that it has high reliability for indicating irreversible worsening, but low sensitivity over short (2-year) periods,[225] as the median time to reach this level is between 15 and 20 years from diagnosis.[301,302]

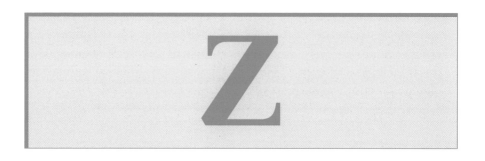

Zanaflex see *Tizanidine.*

Zovirax see *Acyclovir.*

References

1 McArthur JC. Neurologic manifestations of AIDS. Medicine (Baltimore) 1987; 66: 407–37.
2 Petito CK, Navia BA, Cho ES et al. Vacuolar myelopathy pathologically resembling subacute combined degeneration in patients with acquired immunodeficiency syndrome. N Engl J Med 1986; 312: 874–9.
3 Miller DH, Albert PS, Barkhof F et al. Guidelines for the use of magnetic resonance techniques in monitoring the treatment of multiple sclerosis. US National MS Society Task Force. Ann Neurol 1996; 39: 6–16.
4 Fazekas F, Barkhof F, Filippi M et al. The contribution of magnetic resonance imaging to the diagnosis of multiple sclerosis. Neurology 1999; 53: 448–56.
5 WHO. ICIDH-2: International Classification of Impairments, Activities and Participation: A manual of dimensions of disablement and functioning. Geneva: World Health Organization, 1997.
6 Kesselring J, Miller DH, Robb SA et al. Acute disseminated encephalomyelitis. MRI findings and the distinction from multiple sclerosis. Brain 1990; 113: 291–302.
7 Triulzi F, Scotti G. Differential diagnosis of multiple sclerosis: contribution of magnetic resonance techniques. J Neurol Neurosurg Psychiatry 1998; 64(Suppl 1): S6–14.
8 Brew B, Sidtis J, Petito CK, Price RW. The neurologic complications of AIDS and human immunodeficiency virus infection. In: Plum F, ed. Advances in Contemporary Neurology. Chapter 1. Philadelphia: Davis, 1988.
9 Hurst EW. Acute haemorrhagic leuco-encephalitis, a previously undefined entity. Med J Australia 1941; 2: 1–6.
10 Raine CS. The neuropathology of multiple sclerosis. In: Raine CS, McFarland HF, Tourtellotte WW, eds. Multiple Sclerosis, clinical and pathogenetic basis. London: Chapman & Hall Medical, 1997: 151–71.
11 Lucchinetti C, Bruck W, Parisi J et al. Heterogeneity of multiple sclerosis lesions: implications for the pathogenesis of demyelination. Ann Neurol 2000; 47: 707–17.
12 Miller DH, Ormerod IEC, Rudge P et al. Early risk of multiple sclerosis following isolated acute syndromes of the brainstem and spinal cord. Ann Neurol 1989; 26: 635–9.
13 Ford B, Tampieri D, Francis G. Long-term follow-up of acute partial transverse myelopathy. Neurology 1992; 42: 250–2.
14 Morrissey SP, Miller DH, Kendall BE et al. The significance of brain magnetic resonance imaging abnormalities at presentation with clinically isolated syndromes suggestive of multiple sclerosis. A 5-year follow-up study. Brain 1993; 116: 135–46.
15 Campi A, Filippi M, Comi G et al. Acute transverse myelopathy: spinal and cranial MR study with clinical follow-up. AJNR 1995; 16: 115–23.
16 Lycke J, Svennerholm B, Hjelmquist E et al. Acyclovir treatment of relapsing-remitting multiple sclerosis. A randomized, placebo-controlled, double-blind study. J Neurol 1996; 243: 214–24.
17 Bech E, Lycke J, Gadeberg P et al. A randomized, double-blind, placebo-controlled MRI study of anti-herpes virus therapy in MS. Neurology 2002; 58: 31–6
18 Hartung HP, Archelos JJ, Zielasek J et al. Circulating adhesion molecules and inflammatory mediators in demyelination: a review. Neurology 1995; 45: S22–32.

19 Dore-Duffy P, Newman W, Balabanov R et al. Circulating, soluble adhesion proteins in cerebrospinal fluid and serum of patients with multiple sclerosis: correlation with clinical activity. Ann Neurol 1995; 37: 55–62.

20 Giovannoni G, Lai M, Thorpe J et al. Longitudinal study of soluble adhesion molecules in multiple sclerosis: correlation with gadolinium enhanced magnetic resonance imaging. Neurology 1997; 48: 1557–65.

21 Hohlfeld R. Biotechnological agents for the immunotherapy of multiple sclerosis. Principles, problems and perspectives. Brain 1997; 120: 865–916.

21A. Alberts B, Bray D, Lewis J et al., eds. Molecular Biology of the Cell 3rd edition. London: Garland Publishing, 1994.

22 Becker CC, Gidal BE, Fleming JO. Immunotherapy in multiple sclerosis, Part 1. Am J Health Syst Pharm 1995; 52: 1985–2000.

23 Kesselring J, Ormerod IEC, Miller DH, de Boulay EPGH, McDonald WI. Magnetic Resonance Imaging in Multiple Sclerosis: An Atlas of Diagnosis and Differential Diagnosis. Stuttgart: Thieme, 1989.

24 Nikoskelainen E. Symptoms, signs and early course of optic neuritis. Acta Ophthalmol 1975; 53: 254–72.

25 Bielekova B, Goodwin B, Richert N et al. Encephalitogenic potential of the myelin basic protein peptide (amino acids 83-99) in multiple sclerosis: results of a phase II clinical trial with an altered peptide ligand. Nat Med 2000; 6: 1167–75.

26 Kappos L, Comi G, Panitch H et al. Induction of a non-encephalitogenic type 2 T helper-cell autoimmune response in multiple sclerosis after administration of an altered peptide ligand in a placebo-controlled, randomized phase II trial. The Altered Peptide Ligand in Relapsing MS Study Group. Nat Med 2000; 6: 1176–82.

27 Canadian. A randomized controlled trial of amantadine in fatigue associated with multiple sclerosis. The Canadian MS Research Group. Can J Neurol Sci 1987; 14: 273–8.

28 Krupp LB, Coyle PK, Doscher C et al. Fatigue therapy in multiple sclerosis: results of a double-blind, randomized, parallel trial of amantadine, pemoline, and placebo. Neurology 1995; 45: 1956–61.

29 Hauser SL, Dawson DM, Lehrich JR et al. Intensive immunosuppression in progressive multiple sclerosis. A randomized, three-arm study of high-dose intravenous cyclophosphamide, plasma exchange, and ACTH. N Engl J Med 1983; 308: 173–80.

30 Paty DW, Willoughby EW, Whitaker J. Assessing the outcome of experimental therapies in multiple sclerosis patients. In: Rudick RA, Goodkin DE, eds. Treatment of Multiple Sclerosis. London: Springer-Verlag, 1992: 47–90.

31 Francis DA, Bain P, Swan AV, Hughes RA. An assessment of disability rating scales used in multiple sclerosis. Arch Neurol 1991; 48: 299–301.

32 Sharrack B, Hughes RA, Soudain S, Dunn G. The psychometric properties of clinical rating scales used in multiple sclerosis. Brain 1999; 122: 141–59.

33 Bever CT, Jr., Anderson PA, Leslie J et al. Treatment with oral 3,4 diaminopyridine improves leg strength in multiple sclerosis patients: results of a randomized, double-blind, placebo-controlled, crossover trial. Neurology 1996; 47: 1457–62.

34 Polman CH, Bertelsmann FW, de Waal R et al. 4-Aminopyridine is superior to 3,4-diaminopyridine in the treatment of patients with multiple sclerosis. Arch Neurol 1994; 51: 1136–9.

35 Sheean GL, Murray NM, Rothwell JC, Miller DH, Thompson AJ. An open-labelled clinical and electrophysiological study of 3,4 diaminopyridine in the treatment of fatigue in multiple sclerosis. Brain 1998; 121: 967–75.

36 Schwid SR, Petrie MD, McDermott MP et al. Quantitative assessment of sustained-release 4-aminopyridine for symptomatic treatment of multiple sclerosis. Neurology 1997; 48: 817–21.

37 Leger OJ, Yednock TA, Tanner L et al. Humanization of a mouse antibody against human alpha-4 integrin: a potential therapeutic for the treatment of multiple sclerosis. Hum Antibodies 1997; 8: 3–16.

38 Kent SJ, Karlik SJ, Rice GP, Horner HC. A monoclonal antibody to alpha 4-integrin

reverses the MR-detectable signs of experimental allergic encephalomyelitis in the guinea pig. J Magn Reson Imaging 1995; 5: 535–40.

39 Tubridy N, Behan PO, Capildeo R et al. The effect of anti-alpha4 integrin antibody on brain lesion activity in MS. The UK Antegren Study Group. Neurology 1999; 53: 466–72.

40 Miller DH, Khan OA, Sheremata WA et al. A controlled trial of natalizumab for relapsing multiple sclerosis. N Engl J Med 2003; 348(1): 15–23.

41 Van Wauwe JP, De Mey JR, Goossens JG. OKT3: a monoclonal anti-human T lymphocyte antibody with potent mitogenic properties. J Immunol 1980; 124: 2708–13.

42 Weinshenker BG, Rice GP, Noseworthy JH et al. The natural history of multiple sclerosis: a geographically based study. 4. Applications to planning and interpretation of clinical therapeutic trials. Brain 1991; 114: 1057–67.

43 Jonker M, van Lambalgen R, Mitchell DJ, Durham SK, Steinman L. Successful treatment of EAE in rhesus monkeys with MHC class II specific monoclonal antibodies. J Autoimmun 1988; 1: 399–414.

44 Losseff NA, Wang L, Lai HM et al. Progressive cerebral atrophy in multiple sclerosis. A serial MRI study. Brain 1996; 119: 2009–19.

45 van Oosten BW, Lai M, Hodgkinson S et al. Treatment of multiple sclerosis with the monoclonal anti-CD4 antibody cM-T412: results of a randomized, double-blind, placebo-controlled, MR-monitored phase II trial. Neurology 1997; 49: 351–7.

46 Hafler DA, Fallis RJ, Dawson DM et al. Immunologic responses of progressive multiple sclerosis patients treated with an anti-T-cell monoclonal antibody, anti-T12. Neurology 1986; 36: 777–84.

47 Rose LM, Richards TL, Peterson J, Petersen R, Alvord EC, Jr. Resolution of CNS lesions following treatment of experimental allergic encephalomyelitis in macaques with monoclonal antibody to the CD18 leukocyte integrin. Mult Scler 1997; 2: 259–66.

48 Bowen JD, Petersdorf SH, Richards TL et al. Phase I study of a humanized anti-CD11/CD18 monoclonal antibody in multiple sclerosis. Clin Pharmacol Ther 1998; 64: 339–46.

49 Sharon J. The major histocompatibility complex and antigen presentation to T cell. In: Sharon J, ed. Basic Immunology. Philadelphia: Williams & Wilkins, 1998: 15–24.

50 Asherson RA, Khamashta MA, Gil A et al. Cerebrovascular disease and antiphospholipid antibodies in systemic lupus erythematosus, lupus-like disease, and the primary antiphospholipid syndrome. Am J Med 1989; 86: 391–9.

51 Scott TF, Hess D, Brillman J. Antiphospholipid antibody syndrome mimicking multiple sclerosis clinically and by magnetic resonance imaging. Arch Intern Med 1994; 154: 917–20.

52 van Oosten BW, Barkhof F, Truyen L et al. Increased MRI activity and immune activation in two multiple sclerosis patients treated with the monoclonal anti-tumor necrosis factor antibody cA2. Neurology 1996; 47: 1531–4.

53 Rodriguez M, Lucchinetti CF. Is apoptotic death of the oligodendrocyte a critical event in the pathogenesis of multiple sclerosis? Neurology 1999; 53: 1615–16.

54 van der Putten JJ, Hobart JC, Freeman JA, Thompson AJ. Measuring change in disability after inpatient rehabilitation: comparison of the responsiveness of the Barthel Index and the Functional Independence Measure. J Neurol Neurosurg Psychiatry 1999; 66: 480–4.

55 Keltner JL, Johnson CA, Spurr JO, Beck RW. Baseline visual field profile of optic neuritis. The experience of the Optic Neuritis Treatment Trial. Arch Ophthalmol 1993; 111: 231–4.

56 Patterson VH, Heron JR. Visual field abnormalities in multiple sclerosis. J Neurol Neurosurg Psychiatry 1980; 43: 205–9.

57 Liu C, Blumhardt LD. Randomised, double blind, placebo controlled study of interferon beta-1a in relapsing-remitting multiple sclerosis analysed by area under disability/time curves. J Neurol Neurosurg Psychiatry 1999; 67: 451–6.

58 Liu C, Blumhardt LD. Benefits of glatiramer acetate on disability in relapsing-

remitting multiple sclerosis. An analysis by area under disability/time curves. The Copolymer 1 Multiple Sclerosis Study Group. J Neurol Sci 2000; 181: 33–7.

59 Bindal AK, Dunsker SB, Tew JM, Jr. Chiari I malformation: classification and management. Neurosurgery 1995; 37: 1069–74.

60 Ashworth B. Preliminary trial of carisoprodol in multiple sclerosis. Practitioner 1964; 192: 540–2.

61 Sloan RL, Sinclair E, Thompson J, Taylor S, Pentland B. Inter-rater reliability of the modified Ashworth Scale for spasticity in hemiplegic patients. Int J Rehabil Res 1992; 15: 158–61.

62 Shibasaki H, McDonald WI, Kuroiwa Y. Racial modification of clinical picture of multiple sclerosis: comparison between British and Japanese patients. J Neurol Sci 1981; 49: 253–71.

63 Kira J, Yamasaki K, Horiuchi I et al. Changes in the clinical phenotypes of multiple sclerosis during the past 50 years in Japan. J Neurol Sci 1999; 166: 53–7.

64 Kira J, Kanai T, Nishimura Y et al. Western versus Asian types of multiple sclerosis: immunogenetically and clinically distinct disorders. Ann Neurol 1996; 40: 569–74.

65 Jersild C, Fog T, Hansen GS et al. Histocompatibility components in multiple sclerosis, with special reference to clinical course. Lancet 1973; ii: 1221–5.

66 Olerup O, Hillert J. HLA class II-associated genetic susceptibility in multiple sclerosis: a critical evaluation. Tissue Antigens 1991; 38: 1–15.

67 Spurkland A, Ronningen KS, Vandvik B, Thorsby E, Vartdal F. HLA-DQA1 and HLA-DQB1 genes may jointly determine susceptibility to develop multiple sclerosis. Hum Immunol 1991; 30: 69–75.

68 Yamasaki K, Horiuchi I, Minohara M et al. HLA-DPB1*0501-associated opticospinal multiple sclerosis: clinical, neuroimaging and immunogenetic studies. Brain 1999; 122: 1689–96.

69 Yamasaki K. [HLA-DPB1*0501-associated opticospinal multiple sclerosis: clinical, neuroimaging and immunogenetic studies]. Fukuoka Igaku Zasshi 2000; 91: 243–5.

70 Oturai A, Larsen F, Ryder LP et al. Linkage and association analysis of susceptibility regions on chromosomes 5 and 6 in 106 Scandinavian sibling pair families with multiple sclerosis. Ann Neurolo 1999; 46: 612–16.

71 Al-Din AS, Al-Saffar M, Siboo R, Behbehani K. Association between HLA-D region epitopes and multiple sclerosis in Arabs. Tissue Antigens 1986; 27: 196–200.

72 Gorodezky C, Najera R, Rangel BE et al. Immunogenetic profile of multiple sclerosis in Mexican. Hum Immunol 1986; 16: 364–74.

73 Naito S, Kuroiwa Y, Itoyama T et al. HLA and Japanese MS. Tissue Antigens 1978; 12: 19–24.

74 Marrosu MG, Muntoni F, Murru MR et al. Sardinian multiple sclerosis is associated with HLA-DR4: a serology and molecular analysis. Neurology 1988; 38: 1749–53.

75 Vartdal F, Sollid LM, Vandvik B, Markussen G, Thorsby E. Patients with multiple sclerosis carry DQB1 genes which encode shared polymorphic amino acid sequences. Hum Immunol 1989; 25: 103–10.

76 Olerup O, Hillert J, Fredrikson S et al. Primarily chronic progressive and relapsing/remitting multiple sclerosis: two immunogenetically distinct disease entities. Proc Natl Acad Sci USA 1989; 86: 7113–17.

77 Hillert J, Gronning M, Nyland H, Link H, Olerup O. An immunogenetic heterogeneity in multiple sclerosis. J Neurol Neurosurg Psychiatry 1992; 55: 887–90.

78 Haegert DG, Francis GS. HLA-DQ polymorphisms do not explain HLA class II associations with multiple sclerosis in two Canadian patient groups. Neurology 1993; 43: 1207–10.

79 McFarland HF, Martin R, McFarlin DE. Genetic influences in mutiple sclerosis. In: Raine CS, McFarland HF, Tourtellotte WW, eds. Multiple Sclerosis. Clinical and pathogenetic basis. London: Chapman & Hall Medical, 1997: 205–19.

80 Compston A. Neurobiology of multiple sclerosis. In: Compston A, Ebers G, Lassmann H, McDonald I, Matthews B, Wekerle H, eds. McApine's Multiple Sclerosis. London: Churchill Livingstone, 1998: 283–321.

81 Losseff NA, Webb SL, O'Riordan JI et al. Spinal cord atrophy and disability in mul-

tiple sclerosis. A new reproducible and sensitive MRI method with potential to monitor disease progression. Brain 1996; 119: 701–8.

82 Losseff NA, Miller DH. Measures of brain and spinal cord atrophy in multiple sclerosis. J Neurol Neurosurg Psychiatry 1998; 64(Suppl 1): S102–5.

83 Stevenson VL, Leary SM, Losseff NA et al. Spinal cord atrophy and disability in MS: a longitudinal study. Neurology 1998; 51: 234–8.

84 Edwards SG, Gong QY, Liu C et al. Infratentorial atrophy on magnetic resonance imaging and disability in multiple sclerosis. Brain 1999; 122: 291–301.

85 Davie CA, Barker GJ, Webb S et al. Persistent functional deficit in multiple sclerosis and autosomal dominant cerebellar ataxia is associated with axon loss. Brain 1995; 118: 1583–92.

86 Dastidar P, Heinonen T, Lehtimaki T et al. Volumes of brain atrophy and plaques correlated with neurological disability in secondary progressive multiple sclerosis. J Neurol Sci 1999; 165: 36–42.

87 Luks TL, Goodkin DE, Nelson SJ et al. A longitudinal study of ventricular volume in early relapsing-remitting multiple sclerosis. Mult Scler 2000; 6: 332–7.

88 Simon JH, Jacobs LD, Campion MK et al. A longitudinal study of brain atrophy in relapsing multiple sclerosis. The Multiple Sclerosis Collaborative Research Group (MSCRG). Neurology 1999; 53: 139–48.

89 Lin X, Blumhardt LD. Inflammation and atrophy in multiple sclerosis: MRI associations with disease course. J Neurol Sci 2001; 189: 99–104.

90 Liu C, Edwards S, Gong Q, Roberts N, Blumhardt LD. Three dimensional MRI estimates of brain and spinal cord atrophy in multiple sclerosis. J Neurol Neurosurg Psychiatry 1999; 66: 323–30.

91 Rudick RA, Fisher E, Lee JC, Duda JT, Simon J. Brain atrophy in relapsing multiple sclerosis: relationship to relapses, EDSS, and treatment with interferon beta-1a. Mult Scler 2000; 6: 365–72.

92 Molyneux PD, Kappos L, Polman C et al. The effect of interferon beta-1b treatment on MRI measures of cerebral atrophy in secondary progressive multiple sclerosis. European Study Group on Interferon beta-1b in secondary progressive multiple sclerosis. Brain 2000; 123: 2256–63.

93 Ferguson B, Matyszak MK, Esiri MM, Perry VH. Axonal damage in acute multiple sclerosis lesions. Brain 1997; 120: 393–9.

94 Trapp BD, Bo L, Mork S, Chang A. Pathogenesis of tissue injury in MS lesions. J Neuroimmunol 1999; 98: 49–56.

95 Rovaris M, Bozzali M, Rodegher M et al. Brain MRI correlates of magnetization transfer imaging metrics in patients with multiple sclerosis. J Neurol Sci 1999; 166: 58–63.

96 van Waesberghe JH, Kamphorst W, De Groot CJ et al. Axonal loss in multiple sclerosis lesions: magnetic resonance imaging insights into substrates of disability. Ann Neurol 1999; 46: 747–54.

97 Werring DJ, Clark CA, Barker GJ, Thompson AJ, Miller DH. Diffusion tensor imaging of lesions and normal-appearing white matter in multiple sclerosis. Neurology 1999; 52: 1626–32.

98 De Stefano N, Matthews PM, Fu L et al. Axonal damage correlates with disability in patients with relapsing-remitting multiple sclerosis. Results of a longitudinal magnetic resonance spectroscopy study. Brain 1998; 121: 1469–77.

99 Fu L, Matthews PM, De Stefano N, Worsley KJ, Narayanan S, Francis GS et al. Imaging axonal damage of normal-appearing white matter in multiple sclerosis. Brain 1998; 121: 103–13.

100 Evangelou N, Esiri MM, Smith S, Palace J, Matthews PM. Quantitative pathological evidence for axonal loss in normal appearing white matter in multiple sclerosis. Ann Neurol 2000; 47: 391–5.

101 McGavern DB, Murray PD, Rivera-Quinones C et al. Axonal loss results in spinal cord atrophy, electrophysiological abnormalities and neurological deficits following demyelination in a chronic inflammatory model of multiple sclerosis. Brain 2000; 123: 519–31.

102 Yudkin PL, Ellison GW, Ghezzi A et al. Overview of azathioprine treatment in multiple sclerosis. Lancet 1991; 338: 1051–5.

103 Van Scoik KG, Johnson CA, Porter WR. The pharmacology and metabolism of the thiopurine drugs 6-mercaptopurine and azathioprine. Drug Metab Rev 1985; 16: 157–74.

104 Shih WW, Ellison GW, Myers LW, Durkos-Smith D, Fahey JL. Locus of selective depression of human natural killer cells by azathioprine. Clin Immunol Immunopathol 1982; 23: 672–81.

105 Caputo D, Zaffaroni M, Ghezzi A, Cazzullo CL. Azathioprine reduces intrathecal IgG synthesis in multiple sclerosis. Acta Neurol Scand 1987; 75: 84–6.

106 Goodkin DE, Bailly RC, Teetzen ML et al. The efficacy of azathioprine in relapsing-remitting multiple sclerosis. Neurology 1991; 41: 20–5.

107 BDMSATG Group. Double-masked trial of azathioprine in multiple sclerosis. British and Dutch Multiple Sclerosis Azathioprine Trial Group. Lancet 1988; 2: 179–83.

108 Ellison GW, Myers LW, Mickey MR et al. A placebo-controlled, randomized, double-masked, variable dosage, clinical trial of azathioprine with and without methylprednisolone in multiple sclerosis. Neurology 1989; 39: 1018–26.

109 Milanese C, La Mantia L, Salmaggi A et al. Double blind controlled randomized study on azathioprine efficacy in multiple sclerosis. Preliminary results. Ital J Neurol Sci 1988; 9: 53–7.

110 Swinburn WR, Liversedge LA. Long-term treatment of multiple sclerosis with azathioprine. J Neurol Neurosurg Psychiatry 1973; 36: 124–6.

111 Rook GA, Ristori G, Salvetti M et al. Bacterial vaccines for the treatment of multiple sclerosis and other autoimmune disorders. *Immunol Today* 2000; 21: 503–8.

112 Ristori G, Giubilei F, Giunti D et al. Myelin basic protein intramolecular spreading without disease progression in a patient with multiple sclerosis. J Neuroimmunol 2000; 110: 240–3.

113 Feldman RG, Kelly-Hayes M, Conomy JP, Foley JM. Baclofen for spasticity in multiple sclerosis. Double-blind crossover and three-year study. Neurology 1978; 28: 1094–8.

114 Becker WJ, Harris CJ, Long ML et al. Long-term intrathecal baclofen therapy in patients with intractable spasticity. Can J Neurol Sci 1995; 22: 208–17.

115 Cartlidge NE, Hudgson P, Weightman D. A comparison of baclofen and diazepam in the treatment of spasticity. J Neurol Sci 1974; 23: 17–24.

116 Roussan M, Terrence C, Fromm G. Baclofen versus diazepam for the treatment of spasticity and long-term follow-up of baclofen therapy. Pharmatherapeutica 1985; 4: 278–84.

117 Courville CB. Concentric sclerosis. In: Vinken PJ, Bruyn GW, eds. Handbook of Clinical Neurology. Amsterdam: North Holland, 1970: 437–51.

118 Barkhof F, Filippi M, Miller DH et al. Comparison of MRI criteria at first presentation to predict conversion to clinically definite multiple sclerosis. Brain 1997; 120: 2059–69.

119 Collin C, Wade DT, Davies S, Horne V. The Barthel ADL Index: a reliability study. Int Disabil Stud 1988; 10: 61–3.

120 Mahoney FI, Barthel DW. Functional evaluation: the Barthel index. Maryland State Med J 1965; 14: 61–5.

121 van Bennekom CA, Jelles F, Lankhorst GJ, Bouter LM. Responsiveness of the rehabilitation activities profile and the Barthel index. J Clin Epidemiol 1996; 49: 39–44.

122 Beck. An inventory for measuring depression. Arch Gen Psychiatry 1961; 4: 561–71.

123 Sullivan MJ, Weinshenker B, Mikail S, Bishop SR. Screening for major depression in the early stages of multiple sclerosis. Can J Neurol Sci 1995; 22: 228–31.

124 O'Duffy JD, Goldstein NP. Neurologic involvement in seven patients with Behcet's disease. Am J Med 1976; 61: 170–8.

125 Motomura S, Tabira T, Kuroiwa Y. A clinical comparative study of multiple sclerosis and neuro-Behcet's syndrome. J Neurol Neurosurg Psychiatry 1980; 43: 210–13.

126 Morrissey SP, Miller DH, Hermaszewski R et al. Magnetic resonance imaging of the central nervous system in Behcet's disease. Eur Neurol 1993; 33: 287–93.

127 Lublin FD, Reingold SC. Defining the clinical course of multiple sclerosis: results of an international survey. National Multiple Sclerosis Society (USA) Advisory Committee on Clinical Trials of New Agents in Multiple Sclerosis. Neurology 1996; 46: 907–11.

128 Yeung CK, Wong KL, Wong WS, Chan KH. Beta 2-microglobulin and systemic lupus erythematosus. J Rheumatol 1986; 13: 1053–8.

129 Us O, Lolli F, Baig S, Link H. Intrathecal synthesis of beta-2-microglobulin in multiple sclerosis and aseptic meningo-encephalitis. Acta Neurol Scand 1989; 80: 598–602.

130 van Walderveen MA, Kamphorst W, Scheltens P et al. Histopathologic correlate of hypointense lesions on T1-weighted spin-echo MRI in multiple sclerosis. Neurology 1998; 50: 1282–8.

131 van Waesberghe JH, Castelijns JA, Scheltens P et al. Comparison of four potential MR parameters for severe tissue destruction in multiple sclerosis lesions. Magn Reson Imaging 1997; 15: 155–62.

132 Truyen L, van Waesberghe JH, van Walderveen MA et al. Accumulation of hypointense lesions ("black holes") on T1 spin-echo MRI correlates with disease progression in multiple sclerosis. Neurology 1996; 47: 1469–76.

133 Simon JH, Lull J, Jacobs LD et al. A longitudinal study of T1 hypointense lesions in relapsing MS: MSCRG trial of interferon beta-1a. Multiple Sclerosis Collaborative Research Group. Neurology 2000; 55: 185–92.

134 Molyneux PD, Brex PA, Fogg C et al. The precision of T1 hypointense lesion volume quantification in multiple sclerosis treatment trials: a multicenter study. Mult Scler 2000; 6: 237–40.

135 van Poppel H, Vereecken RL, Leruitte A. Neuro-muscular dysfunction of the lower urinary tract in multiple sclerosis. Paraplegia 1983; 21: 374–9.

136 Betts CD, O'Mellow MT, Fowler C. Urinary symptoms and the neurological features of bladder dysfunction in multiple sclerosis. J Neurol Neurosurg Psychiatry 1993; 56: 245–50.

137 Awad SA, Gajewski JB, Sogbein SK, Murray TJ, Field CA. Relationship between neurological and urological status in patients with multiple sclerosis. J Urol 1984; 132: 499–502.

138 Koldewijn EL, Hommes OR, Lemmens WAJG, Debruyne FM, van Kerrebroek PEV. Relationship between lower urinary tract abnormalities and disease related parameters in multiple sclerosis. J Urol 1995; 154: 169–73.

139 McFarland HF. The lesion in multiple sclerosis: clinical, pathological, and magnetic resonance imaging considerations. J Neurol Neurosurg Psychiatry 1998; 64(Suppl 1): S26–30.

140 Samijn JPA, Schipperus MR, van Doorn PA. T-cell depleted autologous bone marrow transplantation for multiple sclerosis: transplantation toxicity and early results in three patients. J Neurol 1999; 246: 1/36–1/37.

141 Snow BJ, Tsui JK, Bhatt MH et al. Treatment of spasticity with botulinum toxin: a double-blind study. Ann Neurol 1990; 28: 512–15.

142 Borg-Stein J, Pine ZM, Miller JR, Brin MF. Botulinum toxin for the treatment of spasticity in multiple sclerosis. New observations. Am J Phys Med Rehabil 1993; 72: 364–8.

143 Hyman N, Barnes M, Bhakta B et al. Botulinum toxin (Dysport) treatment of hip adductor spasticity in multiple sclerosis: a prospective, randomised, double blind, placebo controlled, dose ranging study. J Neurol Neurosurg Psychiatry 2000; 68: 707–12.

144 Hinds JP, Eidelman BH, Wald A. Prevalence of bowel dysfunction in multiple sclerosis. A population survey. Gastroenterology 1990; 98: 1538–42.

145 Chia YW, Fowler CJ, Kamm MA et al. Prevalence of bowel dysfunction in patients with multiple sclerosis and bladder dysfunction. J Neurol 1993; 242: 105–8.

146 Goodkin DE, Hertsgaard D, Seminary J. Upper extremity function in multiple sclerosis: improving assessment sensitivity with box-and-block and nine-hole peg tests. Arch Phys Med Rehabil 1988; 69: 850–4.

147 Chiappa KH. Pattern shift visual, brainstem auditory, and short-latency somatosensory evoked potentials in multiple sclerosis. Neurology 1980; 30: 110–23.

148 Comi G, Leocani L, Medaglini S et al. Measuring evoked responses in multiple sclerosis. Mult Scler 1999; 5: 263–7.

149 Baum K, Scheuler W, Hegerl U, Girke W, Schorner W. Detection of brainstem lesions in multiple sclerosis: comparison of brainstem auditory evoked potentials with nuclear magnetic resonance imaging. Acta Neurol Scand 1988; 77: 283–8.

150 Comi G, Martinelli V, Medaglini S et al. Correlation between multimodal evoked potentials and magnetic resonance imaging in multiple sclerosis. J Neurol 1989; 236: 4–8.

151 Mumford CJ, Compston A. Problems with rating scales for multiple sclerosis: a novel approach – the CAMBS score. J Neurol 1993; 240: 209–15.

152 Sharrack B, Hughes RA. Clinical scales for multiple sclerosis. J Neurol Sci 1996; 135: 1–9.

153 Moreau T, Coles A, Wing M et al. Transient increase in symptoms associated with cytokine release in patients with multiple sclerosis. Brain 1996; 119: 225–37.

154 Coles AJ, Wing MG, Molyneux P et al. Monoclonal antibody treatment exposes three mechanisms underlying the clinical course of multiple sclerosis. Ann Neurol 1999; 46: 296–304.

155 Paolillo A, Coles AJ, Molyneux PD et al. Quantitative MRI in patients with secondary progressive MS treated with monoclonal antibody Campath 1H. Neurology 1999; 53: 751–7.

156 Consroe P, Musty R, Rein J, Tillery W, Pertwee R. The perceived effects of smoked cannabis on patients with multiple sclerosis. Eur Neurol 1997; 38: 44–8.

157 Baker D, Pryce G, Croxford JL et al. Cannabinoids control spasticity and tremor in a multiple sclerosis model. Nature 2000; 404: 84–7.

158 Ungerleider JT, Andyrsiak T, Fairbanks L, Ellison GW, Myers LW. Delta-9-THC in the treatment of spasticity associated with multiple sclerosis. Adv Alcohol Subst Abuse 1987; 7: 39–50.

159 Clifford DB. Tetrahydrocannabinol for tremor in multiple sclerosis. Ann Neurol 1983; 13: 669–71.

160 Killestein J, Hoogervorst EL, Reif M et al. Safety, tolerability, and efficacy of orally administered cannabinoids in MS. Neurology 2002; 58: 1404–7.

161 Hooge JP, Redekop WK. Trigeminal neuralgia in multiple sclerosis. Neurology 1995; 45: 1294–6.

162 Sechi GP, Zuddas M, Piredda M et al. Treatment of cerebellar tremors with carbamazepine: a controlled trial with long-term follow-up. Neurology 1989; 39: 1113–15.

163 Kuby J. Overview of the immune system. In: Kuby J, ed. Immunology. New York: W. H. Freeman and Company, 1997: 47–83.

164 Brown JH, Jardetzky TS, Gorga JC et al. Three-dimensional structure of the human class II histocompatibility antigen HLA-DR1. Nature 1993; 364: 33–9.

165 Zamvil SS, Steinman L. The T lymphocyte in experimental allergic encephalomyelitis. Annu Rev Immunol 1990; 8: 579–621.

166 O'Neill JK, Baker D, Davison AN et al. Control of immune-mediated disease of the central nervous system with monoclonal (CD4-specific) antibodies. J Neuroimmunol 1993; 45: 1–14.

167 Abbas AK, Murphy KM, Sher A. Functional diversity of helper T lymphocytes. Nature 1996; 383: 787–93.

168 Lindsey JW, Hodgkinson S, Mehta R et al. Repeated treatment with chimeric anti-CD4 antibody in multiple sclerosis. Ann Neurol 1994; 36: 183–9.

169 Rep MH, van Oosten BW, Roos MT et al. Treatment with depleting CD4 monoclonal antibody results in a preferential loss of circulating naive T cells but does not affect IFN-gamma secreting TH1 cells in humans. J Clin Invest 1997; 99: 2225–31.

170 Crucian B, Dunne P, Friedman H et al. Alterations in levels of CD28-/CD8+ suppressor cell precursor and CD45RO+/CD4+ memory T lymphocytes in the peripheral blood of multiple sclerosis patients. Clin Diagn Lab Immunol 1995; 2: 249–52.

171 McCallum K, Esiri MM, Tourtellotte WW, Booss J. T cell subsets in multiple sclerosis.

Gradients at plaque borders and differences in nonplaque regions. Brain 1987; 110: 1297–308.

172 Lucchinetti CF, Rodriguez M. The controversy surrounding the pathogenesis of the multiple sclerosis lesion. Mayo Clin Proc 1997; 72: 665–78.

173 Ganes T. Somatosensory evoked responses and central afferent conduction times in patients with multiple sclerosis. J Neurol Neurosurg Psychiatry 1980; 43: 948–53.

174 Hess CW, Mills KR, Murray NM, Schriefer TN. Magnetic brain stimulation: central motor conduction studies in multiple sclerosis. Ann Neurol 1987; 22: 744–52.

175 Jones SM, Streletz LJ, Raab VE, Knobler RL, Lublin FD. Lower extremity motor evoked potentials in multiple sclerosis. Arch Neurol 1991; 48: 944–8.

176 Ravnborg M, Liguori R, Christiansen P, Larsson H, Sorensen PS. The diagnostic reliability of magnetically evoked motor potentials in multiple sclerosis. Neurology 1992; 42: 1296–301.

177 Brain WR, Wilkinson M. The association of cervical spondylosis and disseminated sclerosis. Brain 1957; 80: 456–78.

178 Jacobs LD, Beck RW, Simon JH et al. Intramuscular interferon beta-1a therapy initiated during a first demyelinating event in multiple sclerosis. CHAMPS Study Group. N Engl J Med 2000; 343: 898–904.

179 Prineas JW, Barnard RO, Revesz T et al. Multiple sclerosis. Pathology of recurrent lesions. Brain 1993; 116: 681–93.

180 Raine CS. Demyelinating diseases. In: Davis RL, Robertson DM, eds. Textbook of Neuropathology. New York: Williams and Wilkins, 1997: 627–714.

181 Trapp BD, Peterson J, Ransohoff RM et al. Axonal transection in the lesions of multiple sclerosis. N Engl J Med 1998; 338: 278–85.

182 Mews I, Bergmann M, Bunkowski S, Gullotta F, Bruck W. Oligodendrocyte and axon pathology in clinically silent multiple sclerosis lesions. Mult Scler 1998; 4: 55–62.

183 Lucchinetti C, Bruck W, Parisi J et al. A quantitative analysis of oligodendrocytes in multiple sclerosis lesions. A study of 113 cases. Brain 1999; 122: 2279–95.

184 Wolswijk G. Oligodendrocyte survival, loss and birth in lesions of chronic-stage multiple sclerosis. Brain 2000; 123: 105–15.

185 Beutler E. Cladribine (2-chlorodeoxyadenosine). Lancet 1992; 340: 952–6.

186 Sipe JC, Romine JS, Koziol JA et al. Cladribine in treatment of chronic progressive multiple sclerosis. Lancet 1994; 344: 9–13.

187 Rice GP, Filippi M, Comi G. Cladribine and progressive MS: clinical and MRI outcomes of a multicenter controlled trial. Cladribine MRI Study Group. Neurology 2000; 54: 1145–55

188 Kita M, Goodkin D. Treatments for progressive forms of MS. In: Hawkins CP, Wolinsky JS, eds. Principles of Treatments in Multiple Sclerosis. Oxford: Butterworth Heinemann, 2000: 148–61.

189 Schumacher GA, Beebe G, Kebler RF et al. Problems of experimental trials of therapy in multiple sclerosis: report by the panel on the evaluation of experimental trials of therapy in multiple sclerosis. Ann NY Acad Sci 1965; 122: 552–68.

190 McDonald WI, Halliday AM. Diagnosis and classification of multiple sclerosis. Br Med Bull 1977; 33: 4–9.

191 Poser CM, Paty DW, Scheinberg L et al. New diagnostic criteria for multiple sclerosis: guidelines for research protocols. Ann Neurol 1983; 13: 227–31.

192 McDonald WI, Compston A, Edan G et al. Recommended diagnostic criteria for multiple sclerosis: Guidelines from the International Panel on the Diagnosis of Multiple Sclerosis. Ann Neurol 2001; 50: 121–7.

193 Tintore M, Rovira A, Martinez MJ et al. Isolated demyelinating syndromes: comparison of different MR imaging criteria to predict conversion to clinically definite multiple sclerosis. AJNR 2000; 21: 702–6.

194 Link H, Tibbling G. Principles of albumin and IgG analyses in neurological disorders. III. Evaluation of IgG synthesis within the central nervous system in multiple sclerosis. Scand J Clin Lab Invest 1977; 37: 397–401.

195 Andersson M, Alvarez-Cermeno J, Bernardi G et al. Cerebrospinal fluid in the diag-

nosis of multiple sclerosis: a consensus report. J Neurol Neurosurg Psychiatry 1994; 57: 897–902.

196 Halliday AM. Evoked potential in clinical testing. London: Churchill Livingstone, 1993.

197 Rizzo JF, Lessell S. Risk of developing multiple sclerosis after uncomplicated optic neuritis: a long term perspective study. Neurology 1988; 38: 185–90.

198 Group TONS. The five-year risk of multiple sclerosis after optic neuritis: experience of the optic neuritis treatment trial. Neurology 1997; 49: 1404–13.

199 Sailer M, O'Riordan JI, Thompson AJ et al. Quantitative MRI in patients with clinically isolated syndromes suggestive of demyelination. Neurology 1999; 52: 599–606.

200 Riise T. Cluster studies in multiple sclerosis. Neurology 1997; 49(Suppl 2): S27–32.

201 Poser CM, Benedikz J, Hibberd PL. The epidemiology of multiple sclerosis: the Iceland model. Onset-adjusted prevalence rate and other methodological considerations. J Neurol Sci 1992; 111: 143–52.

202 Peyser JM, Rao SM, LaRocca NG, Kaplan E. Guidelines for neuropsychological research in multiple sclerosis. Arch Neurol 1990; 47: 94–7.

203 Beatty WW, Goodkin DE, Monson N, Beatty PA. Cognitive disturbances in patients with relapsing remitting multiple sclerosis. Arch Neurol 1989; 46: 1113–19.

204 Rao SM, Leo GJ, Bernardin L, Unverzagt F. Cognitive dysfunction in multiple sclerosis. I. Frequency, patterns, and prediction. Neurology 1991; 41: 685–91.

205 Comi G, Filippi M, Martinelli V et al. Brain MRI correlates of cognitive impairment in primary and secondary progressive multiple sclerosis. J Neurol Sci 1995; 132: 222–7.

206 Kujala P, Portin R, Ruutiainen J. The progress of cognitive decline in multiple sclerosis. A controlled 3-year follow-up. Brain 1997; 120: 289–97.

207 Beatty WW, Goodkin DE, Monson N, Beatty PA, Hertsgaard D. Anterograde and retrograde amnesia in patients with chronic progressive multiple sclerosis. Arch Neurol 1988; 45: 611–19.

208 Litvan I, Grafman J, Vendrell P, Martinez JM. Slowed information processing in multiple sclerosis. Arch Neurol 1988; 45: 281–5.

209 Peyser JM, Edwards KR, Poser CM, Filskov SB. Cognitive function in patients with multiple sclerosis. Arch Neurol 1980; 37: 577–9.

210 Heaton RK, Nelson LM, Thompson DS, Burks JS, Franklin GM. Neuropsychological findings in relapsing-remitting and chronic progressive multiple sclerosis. J Consult Clin Psychol 1985; 53: 103–10.

211 Prosiegel M., Michael C. Neuropsychology and multiple sclerosis: diagnostic and rehabilitative approaches. J Neurol Sci 1993; 115(Suppl): S51–S54.

212 Minden SL, Schiffer RB. Affective disorders in multiple sclerosis. Arch Neurol 1990; 47: 98–104.

213 Li DK, Paty DW. Magnetic resonance imaging results of the PRISMS trial: a randomized, double-blind, placebo-controlled study of interferon-beta1a in relapsing-remitting multiple sclerosis. Prevention of Relapses and Disability by Interferon-beta1a Subcutaneously in Multiple Sclerosis. Ann Neurol 1999; 46: 197–206.

214 Jans H, Heltberg A, Zeeberg I et al. Immune complexes and the complement factors C4 and C3 in cerebrospinal fluid and serum from patients with chronic progressive multiple sclerosis. *Acta Neurol Scand* 1984; 69: 34–8.

215 Sanders ME, Koski CL, Robbins D et al. Activated terminal complement in cerebrospinal fluid in Guillain-Barre syndrome and multiple sclerosis. J Immunol 1986; 136: 4456–9.

216 Compston DA, Morgan BP, Campbell AK et al. Immunocytochemical localization of the terminal complement complex in multiple sclerosis. Neuropathol Appl Neurobiol 1989; 15: 307–16.

217 Sellebjerg F, Christiansen M, Garred P. MBP, anti-MBP and anti-PLP antibodies, and intrathecal complement activation in multiple sclerosis. Mult Scler 1998; 4: 127–31.

218 Calida DM, Constantinescu C, Purev E et al. Cutting edge: C3, a key component of complement activation, is not required for the development of myelin oligodendrocyte glycoprotein peptide-induced experimental autoimmune encephalomyelitis in mice. J Immunol 2001; 166: 723–6.

219 Revel MP, Valiente E, Gray F et al. Concentric MR patterns in multiple sclerosis. Report of two cases. J Neuroradiol 1993; 20: 252–7.

220 Sadovnick AD, Armstrong H, Rice GP et al. A population-based study of multiple sclerosis in twins: update. Ann Neurol 1993; 33: 281–5.

221 Rasminsky M, Sears TA. Internodal conduction in undissected demyelinated nerve fibres. J Physiol 1972; 227: 323–50.

222 Rudick RA. Clinical outcomes assessment in multiple sclerosis: Part I. Mult Scler 1996; 2: 244–6.

223 Myers LW, Ellison GW, Leake BD, Mickey MR. Selection of patients for therapeutic clinical trials in multiple sclerosis. In: Siva A, Kesselring J, Thompson AJ, eds. Frontiers in Multiple Sclerosis. London: Martin Dunitz, 1999: 151–93.

224 Weinshenker BG, Issa M, Baskerville J. Meta-analysis of the placebo-treated groups in clinical trials of progressive MS. Neurology 1996; 46: 1613–19.

225 Liu C, Blumhardt LD. Disability outcome measures in therapeutic trials of relapsing-remitting multiple sclerosis: effects of heterogeneity of disease course in placebo cohorts. J Neurol Neurosurg Psychiatry 2000; 68: 450–7.

226 Cronbach LJ, Meehl PE. Construct validity in psychological tests. Psychol Bull 1955; 52: 281–302.

227 Beck RW, Ruchman MC, Savino PJ, Schatz NJ. Contrast sensitivity measurements in acute and resolved optic neuritis. Br J Ophthalmol 1984; 68: 756–9.

228 Fleishman JA, Beck RW, Linares OA, Klein JW. Deficits in visual function after resolution of optic neuritis. Ophthalmology 1987; 94: 1029–35.

229 Trobe JD, Beck RW, Moke PS, Cleary PA. Contrast sensitivity and other vision tests in the optic neuritis treatment trial. Am J Ophthalmol 1996; 121: 547–53.

230 Folstein MF, Folstein SE, McHugh PR. "Mini-mental state". A practical method for grading the cognitive state of patients for the clinician. J Psychiatr Res 1975; 12: 189–98.

231 Wechsler D. Wechsler Adult Intelligence Scale – Revised. New York: Psychological Corporation, 1981.

232 Gronwall DM. Paced auditory serial-addition task: a measure of recovery from concussion. Percept Mot Skills 1977; 44: 367–73.

233 Smith A. Symbol Digit Modalities Test: Manual. Los Angeles: Western Psychological Services, 1982.

234 Rao SM, Hammeke TA, McQuillen MP, Khatri BO, Lloyd D. Memory disturbance in chronic progressive multiple sclerosis. Arch Neurol 1984; 41: 625–31.

235 Wechsler D. Wechsler Adult Intelligence Scale – Revised. San Antonio: Psychological Corporation, 1987.

236 Benton A. Differential behavioral effects in frontal lobe disease. Neuropsychologia 1968; 6: 53–60.

237 Kaplan E, Goodglass H, Weintraub S. Boston Naming Test. Philadelphia: Lea & Febiger, 1983.

238 Heaton RK. Wisconsin Card Sorting Test Manual. Odessa, FL: Psychological Assessment Resources, 1981.

239 Beatty W. Assessment of cognitive and psychological functions in patients with multiple sclerosis: considerations for databasing. Mult Scler 1999; 5: 239–43.

240 Simon JH, Holtas SL, Schiffer RB et al. Corpus callosum and subcallosal-periventricular lesions in multiple sclerosis: detection with MR. Radiology 1986; 160: 363–7.

241 Gean-Marton AD, Vezina LG, Marton K et al. Abnormal corpus callosum: a sensitive and specific indicator of multiple sclerosis. Radiology 1991; 180: 215–21.

242 Barnard RO, Triggs M. Corpus callosum in multiple sclerosis. J Neurol Neurosurg Psychiatry 1974; 37: 1259–64.

243 Pelletier J, Habib M, Lyon-Caen O et al. Functional and magnetic resonance imaging correlates of callosal involvement in multiple sclerosis. Arch Neurol 1993; 50: 1077–82.

244 Palmer S, Bradley WG, Chen DY, Patel S. Subcallosal striations: early findings of multiple sclerosis on sagittal, thin-section, fast FLAIR MR images. Radiology 1999; 210: 149–53.

245 Kidd D, Barkhof F, McConnell R et al. Cortical lesions in multiple sclerosis. Brain 1999; 122: 17–26.

246 Jeffery DR, Absher J, Pfeiffer FE, Jackson H. Cortical deficits in multiple sclerosis on the basis of subcortical lesions. Mult Scler 2000; 6: 50–5.

247 Lazeron RH, Langdon DW, Filippi M et al. Neuropsychological impairment in multiple sclerosis patients: the role of (juxta)cortical lesion on FLAIR. Mult Scler 2000; 6: 280–5.

248 Filippi M, Yousry T, Baratti C et al. Quantitative assessment of MRI lesion load in multiple sclerosis. A comparison of conventional spin-echo with fast fluid-attenuated inversion recovery. Brain 1996; 119: 1349–55.

249 Bastianello S, Bozzao A, Paolillo A et al. Fast spin-echo and fast fluid-attenuated inversion-recovery versus conventional spin-echo sequences for MR quantification of multiple sclerosis lesions. AJNR 1997; 18: 699–704.

250 Gawne-Cain ML, O'Riordan JI, Thompson AJ, Moseley IF, Miller DH. Multiple sclerosis lesion detection in the brain: a comparison of fast fluid-attenuated inversion recovery and conventional T2-weighted dual spin echo. Neurology 1997; 49: 364–70.

251 Kaufman DI, Trobe JD, Eggenberger ER, Whitaker JN. Practice parameter: the role of corticosteroids in the management of acute monosymptomatic optic neuritis. Report of the Quality Standards Subcommittee of the American Academy of Neurology. Neurology 2000; 54: 2039–44.

252 Sharrack B, Hughes RA, Morris RW et al. The effect of oral and intravenous methylprednisolone treatment on subsequent relapse rate in multiple sclerosis. J Neurol Sci 2000; 173: 73–7.

253 Sellebjerg F, Frederiksen JL, Nielsen PM, Olesen J. Double-blind, randomized, placebo-controlled study of oral, high-dose methylprednisolone in attacks of MS. Neurology 1998; 51: 529–34.

254 Burnham JA, Wright RR, Dreisbach J, Murray RS. The effect of high-dose steroids on MRI gadolinium enhancement in acute demyelinating lesions. Neurology 1991; 41: 1349–54.

255 Barkhof F, Frequin ST, Hommes OR et al. A correlative triad of gadolinium-DTPA MRI, EDSS, and CSF-MBP in relapsing multiple sclerosis patients treated with high-dose intravenous methylprednisolone. Neurology 1992; 42: 63–7.

256 Miller DH, Thompson AJ, Morrissey SP et al. High dose steroids in acute relapses of multiple sclerosis: MRI evidence for a possible mechanism of therapeutic effect. J Neurol Neurosurg Psychiatry 1992; 55: 450–3.

257 Cronstein BN, Kimmel SC, Levin RI, Martiniuk F, Weissmann G. A mechanism for the antiinflammatory effects of corticosteroids: the glucocorticoid receptor regulates leukocyte adhesion to endothelial cells and expression of endothelial-leukocyte adhesion molecule 1 and intercellular adhesion molecule 1. Proc Natl Acad Sci USA 1992; 89: 9991–5.

258 Boumpas DT, Paliogianni F, Anastassiou ED, Balow JE. Glucocorticosteroid action on the immune system: molecular and cellular aspects. Clin Exp Rheumatol 1991; 9: 413–23.

259 AyanlarBatuman O, Ferrero AP, Diaz A, Jimenez SA. Regulation of transforming growth factor-beta 1 gene expression by glucocorticoids in normal human T lymphocytes. J Clin Invest 1991; 88: 1574–80.

260 Polman CH, van der Wiel HE, Netelenbos JC, Teule GJ, Koetsier JC. A commentary on steroid treatment in multiple sclerosis. Arch Neurol 1991; 48: 1011–2.

261 Tourtellotte WW, Potvin AR, Fleming JO et al. Multiple sclerosis: measurement and validation of central nervous system IgG synthesis rate. Neurology 1980; 30: 240–4.

262 Reiber H. Flow rate of cerebrospinal fluid (CSF) – a concept common to normal blood-CSF barrier function and to dysfunction in neurological diseases. J Neurol Sci 1994; 122: 189–203.

263 Hafler DA, Orav J, Gertz R, Stazzone L, Weiner HL. Immunologic effects of cyclophosphamide/ACTH in patients with chronic progressive multiple sclerosis. J Neuroimmunol 1991; 32: 149–58.

264 Moody DJ, Kagan J, Liao D, Ellison GW, Myers LW. Administration of monthly-pulse cyclophosphamide in multiple sclerosis patients. Effects of long-term treatment on immunologic parameters. J Neuroimmunol 1987; 14: 161–73.

265 Lamers KJ, Uitdehaag BM, Hommes OR et al. The short-term effect of an immunosuppressive treatment on CSF myelin basic protein in chronic progressive multiple sclerosis. J Neurol Neurosurg Psychiatry 1988; 51: 1334–7.

266 Weiner HL, Mackin GA, Orav EJ et al. Intermittent cyclophosphamide pulse therapy in progressive multiple sclerosis: final report of the Northeast Cooperative Multiple Sclerosis Treatment Group. Neurology 1993; 43: 910–8.

267 Likosky WH, Fireman B, Elmore R et al. Intense immunosuppression in chronic progressive multiple sclerosis: the Kaiser study. J Neurol Neurosurg Psychiatry 1991; 54: 1055–60.

268 TCCMSG, Group) TCCMS. The Canadian cooperative trial of cyclophosphamide and plasma exchange in progressive multiple sclerosis. The Canadian Cooperative Multiple Sclerosis Study Group. Lancet 1991; 337: 441–6.

269 Rudge P, Koetsier JC, Mertin J et al. Randomised double blind controlled trial of cyclosporin in multiple sclerosis. J Neurol Neurosurg Psychiatry 1989; 52: 559–65.

270 MSSG. Efficacy and toxicity of cyclosporine in chronic progressive multiple sclerosis: a randomized, double-blinded, placebo-controlled clinical trial. The Multiple Sclerosis Study Group. Ann Neurol 1990; 27: 591–605.

271 Coyle PK. The neuroimmunology of multiple sclerosis. Adv Neuroimmunol 1996; 6: 143–54.

272 Raine CS. Multiple sclerosis: immune system molecule expression in the central nervous system. J Neuropathol Exp Neurol 1994; 53: 328–37.

273 Barnes M. Management of spasticity – pharmacological agents. In: Hawkins CP, Wolinsky JS, eds. Principles of Treatments in Multiple Sclerosis. Oxford: Butterworth Heinemann, 2000: 184–200.

274 Hallpike JF, Adams CWM, Tourtelotte WW. Multiple Sclerosis: Pathology, Diagnosis and Management. Baltimore: Williams & Wilkins, 1983: 231–5.

275 Horowitz AL, Kaplan RD, Grewe G, White RT, Salberg LM. The ovoid lesion: a new MR observation in patients with multiple sclerosis. AJNR 1989; 10: 303–5.

276 Joffe RT, Lippert GP, Gray TA, Sawa G, Horvath Z. Mood disorder and multiple sclerosis. Arch Neurol 1987; 44: 376–8.

277 Minden SL, Orav J, Reich P. Depression in multiple sclerosis. Gen Hosp Psychiatry 1987; 9: 426–34.

278 Surridge D. An investigation into some psychiatric aspects of multiple sclerosis. Br J Psychiatry 1969; 115: 749–64.

279 Whitlock FA, Siskind MM. Depression as a major symptom of multiple sclerosis. J Neurol Neurosurg Psychiatry 1980; 43: 861–5.

280 Pujol J, Bello J, Deus J, Marti-Vilalta JL, Capdevila A. Lesions in the left arcuate fasciculus region and depressive symptoms in multiple sclerosis. Neurology 1997; 49: 1105–10.

281 Youl BD, Kermode AG, Thompson AJ et al. Destructive lesions in demyelinating disease. J Neurol Neurosurg Psychiatry 1991; 54: 288–92.

282 Philp T., Read D.J., Higson R.H. The urodynamic characteristics of multiple sclerosis. Br J Urol 1981; 53: 672–5.

283 Petersen T, Pedersen E. Neurourodynamic evaluation of voiding dysfunction in multiple sclerosis. Acta Neurol Scand 1984; 69: 402–11.

284 McGuire EJ, Savastano JA. Urodynamic findings and long-term outcome management of patients with multiple sclerosis-induced lower urinary tract dysfunction. J Urol 1984; 132: 713–15.

285 Weinstein MS, Cardenas DD, O'Shaughnessy EJ, Catanzaro ML. Carbon dioxide cystometry and postural changes in patients with multiple sclerosis. Arch Phys Med Rehabil 1988; 69: 923–7.

286 Litwiller SE, Frohman EM, Zimmern PE. Multiple sclerosis and the urologist. J Urol 1999; 161: 743–57.

287   Blaivas JG, Bhimani G, Labib KB. Vesicourethral dysfunction in multiple sclerosis. J Urol 1979; 22: 342–7.

288   Goldstein I, Siroky MB, Sax DS, Krane RJ. Neurourologic abnormalities in multiple sclerosis. J Urol 1982; 128: 541–5.

289   Devic E. Myelite subaigue compliquée de nevrite optique. Bull Med (Paris) 1894; 8: 1033.

290   Hickey WF. The pathology of multiple sclerosis: a historical perspective. J Neuroimmunol 1999; 98: 37–44.

291   Kesselring J, Miller DH. Differential diagnosis. In: Miller DH, Kesselring J, McDonald WI, Paty DW, Thompson AJ, eds. Magnetic Resonance in Multiple Sclerosis. Cambridge: Cambridge University Press, 1997: 63–107.

292   Lauer K. The risk of multiple sclerosis in the U.S.A. in relation to sociogeographic features: a factor-analytic study. J Clin Epidemiol 1994; 47: 43–8.

293   Tola MR, Granieri E, Malagu S et al. Dietary habits and multiple sclerosis. A retrospective study in Ferrara, Italy. Acta Neurol (Napoli) 1994; 16: 189–97.

294   Horsfield MA, Larsson HB, Jones DK, Gass A. Diffusion magnetic resonance imaging in multiple sclerosis. J Neurol Neurosurg Psychiatry 1998; 64(Suppl 1): S80–4.

295   Larsson HB, Thomsen C, Frederiksen J, Stubgaard M, Henriksen O. In vivo magnetic resonance diffusion measurement in the brain of patients with multiple sclerosis. Magn Reson Imaging 1992; 10: 7–12.

296   Wilson M, Morgan PS, Lin X, Turner BP, Blumhardt LD. Quantitative diffusion weighted magnetic resonance imaging, cerebral atrophy, and disability in multiple sclerosis. J Neurol Neurosurg Psychiatry 2001; 70: 318–22.

297   Bauer HJ, Hanefield FA. Multiple Sclerosis. Its impact from childhood to old age. London: Saunders, 1993.

298   Lhermitte F, Mateau R, Gazengel J et al. The frequency of relapse in multiple sclerosis: a study based on 245 cases. J Neurology 1973; 205: 407–59.

299   Kurtzke JF. Clinical features of multiple sclerosis. In: Vinken PJ, Bruyn GW, eds. Handbook of Clinical Neurology. Amsterdam: Elsevier, 1970: 161–216.

300   WHO. International classification of impairments, disabilities and handicaps. Geneva: World Health Organization, 1980.

301   Weinshenker BG, Bass B, Rice GP et al. The natural history of multiple sclerosis: a geographically based study. I. Clinical course and disability. Brain 1989; 112: 133–46.

302   Runmarker B, Andersen O. Prognostic factors in a multiple sclerosis incidence cohort with twenty-five years of follow-up. Brain 1993; 116: 117–34.

303   Broman T, Andersen O, Bergmann L. Clinical studies on multiple sclerosis. I. Presentation of an incidence material from Gothenburg. Acta Neurol Scand 1981; 63: 6–33.

304   Kurtzke JF. A new scale for evaluating disability in multiple sclerosis. Neurology (Minn.) 1955; 5: 580–3.

305   Kurtzke JF. Rating neurologic impairment in multiple sclerosis: an expanded disability status scale (EDSS). Neurology 1983; 33: 1444–52.

306   Kurtzke JF. On the evaluation of disability in multiple sclerosis. Neurology (Minn.) 1961; 11: 686–94.

307   Sipe JC, Knobler RL, Braheny SL et al. A neurologic rating scale (NRS) for use in multiple sclerosis. Neurology 1984; 34: 1368–72.

308   Mickey MR, Ellison GW, Myers LW. An illness severity score for multiple sclerosis. Neurology 1984; 34: 1343–7.

309   Hohol MJ, Orav EJ, Weiner HL. Disease steps in multiple sclerosis: a simple approach to evaluate disease progression. Neurology 1995; 45: 251–5.

310   Granger CV, Cotter AC, Hamilton BB, Fiedler RC, Hens MM. Functional assessment scales: a study of persons with multiple sclerosis. Arch Phys Med Rehabil 1990; 71: 870–5.

311   Cutter GR, Baier ML, Rudick RA et al. Development of a multiple sclerosis functional composite as a clinical trial outcome measure. Brain 1999; 122: 871–82.

312 Sharrack B, Hughes RA. The Guy's Neurological Disability Scale (GNDS): a new disability measure for multiple sclerosis. Mult Scler 1999; 5: 223–33.

313 International Federation of Multiple Sclerosis Societies. Minimal Record of Disability for Multiple Sclerosis. New York: National Multiple Sclerosis Society of the United States, 1985.

314 Potvin AR, Tourtellotte WW. The neurological examination: advancements in its quantification. Arch Phys Med Rehabil 1975; 56: 425–37.

315 Cook SD, Devereux C, Troiano R et al. Effect of total lymphoid irradiation in chronic progressive multiple sclerosis. Lancet 1986; 1: 1405–9.

316 Geschwind N. Disconnexion syndromes in animals and man. Brain 1965; 88: 237, 585.

317 Rao SM, Bernardin L, Leo GJ et al. Cerebral disconnection in multiple sclerosis: relationship to atrophy of the corpus callosum. Arch Neurol 1989; 46: 918–20.

318 Dietemann JL, Beigelman C, Rumbach L et al. Multiple sclerosis and corpus callosum atrophy: relationship of MRI findings to clinical data. Neuroradiology 1988; 30: 478–80.

319 McAlpine D, Lumsden CE, Acheson ED, eds. Multiple sclerosis: a reappraisal. Baltimore: Williams and Wilkins: 132–96.

320 Poser CM. The epidemiology of multiple sclerosis: a general overview. Ann Neurol 1994; 36(Suppl 2): S180–93.

321 Rodriguez M, Scheithauer B. Ultrastructure of multiple sclerosis. Ultrastruct Pathol 1994; 18: 3–13.

322 Griffin JF, Wray SH. Acquired colour vision defects in retrobulbar neuritis. Am J Ophthalmol 1978; 86: 193–201.

323 Moulin DE, Foley KM, Ebers GC. Pain syndromes in multiple sclerosis. Neurology 1988; 38: 1830–4.

324 Samkoff LM, Daras M, Tuchman AJ, Koppel BS. Amelioration of refractory dysesthetic limb pain in multiple sclerosis by gabapentin. Neurology 1977; 49: 304–5.

325 Kazis LE, Anderson JJ, Meenan RF. Effect sizes for interpreting changes in health status. Med Care 1989; 27: S178–89.

326 Polman CK. Multiple Sclerosis. The guide to treatment and management. New York: Demos, 2001.

327 Bevilacqua MP. Endothelial-leukocyte adhesion molecules. Annu Rev Immunol 1993; 11: 767–804.

328 Giovannoni G, Thorpe JW, Kidd D et al. Soluble E-selectin in multiple sclerosis: raised concentrations in patients with primary progressive disease. J Neurol Neurosurg Psychiatry 1996; 60: 20–6.

329 McDonnell GV, McMillan SA, Douglas JP, Droogan AG, Hawkins SA. Serum soluble adhesion molecules in multiple sclerosis: raised sVCAM-1, sICAM-1 and sE-selectin in primary progressive disease. J Neurol 1999; 246: 87–92.

330 IFNB, Group TIMSS. Interferon beta-1b is effective in relapsing-remitting multiple sclerosis. I. Clinical results of a multicenter, randomized, double- blind, placebo-controlled trial. The IFNB Multiple Sclerosis Study Group. Neurology 1993; 43: 655–61.

331 Jacobs LD, Cookfair DL, Rudick RA et al. Intramuscular interferon beta-1a for disease progression in relapsing multiple sclerosis. The Multiple Sclerosis Collaborative Research Group (MSCRG). Ann Neurol 1996; 39: 285–94.

332 Johnson KP, Brooks BR, Cohen JA et al. Copolymer 1 reduces relapse rate and improves disability in relapsing-remitting multiple sclerosis: results of a phase III multicenter, double-blind placebo-controlled trial. The Copolymer 1 Multiple Sclerosis Study Group. Neurology 1995; 45: 1268–76.

333 PRISMS, Group PoRaDbIb-aSiMSS. Randomised double-blind placebo-controlled study of interferon beta-1a in relapsing/remitting multiple sclerosis. Lancet 1998; 352: 1498–504.

334 Paty DW. Magnetic resonance imaging in the assessment of disease activity in multiple sclerosis. Can J Neurol Sci 1988; 15: 266–72.

335 Kurtzke JF. MS epidemiology world wide. One view of current status. Acta Neurol Scand Suppl 1995; 161: 23–33.

336 Dean G, Kurtzke JF. On the risk of multiple sclerosis according to age at immigration to South Africa. Br Med J 1971; 3: 725–9.

337 Kurtzke JF, Delasnerie-Laupretre N, Wallin MT. Multiple sclerosis in North African migrants to France. Acta Neurol Scand 1998; 98: 302–9.

338 Elian M, Nightingale S, Dean G. Multiple sclerosis among United Kingdom-born children of immigrants from the Indian subcontinent, Africa and the West Indies. J Neurol Neurosurg Psychiatry 1990; 53: 906–11.

339 Kurtzke JF, Hyllested K, Heltberg A. Multiple sclerosis in the Faroe Islands: transmission across four epidemics. Acta Neurol Scand 1995; 91: 321–5.

340 Sadovnick A.D., Ebers G.C. Epidemiology of multiple sclerosis: a critical overview. Can J Neurol Sci 1993; 20: 17–29.

341 MacMahon B. Epidemiological methods. In: Clark DW, MacMahon B, eds. Preventive Medicine. Boston: Little Brown, 1967: 81–104.

342 Kurtzke JF, Hyllested K. Multiple sclerosis: an epidemic disease in the Faroes. Trans Am Neurol Assoc 1975; 100: 213–15.

343 Kurtzke JF, Hyllested K, Heltberg A, Olsen A. Multiple sclerosis in the Faroe Islands. 5. The occurrence of the fourth epidemic as validation of transmission. Acta Neurol Scand 1993; 88: 161–73.

344 Cook SD, Gudmundsson G, Benedikz J, Dowling PC. Multiple sclerosis and distemper in Iceland 1966–1978. Acta Neurol Scand 1980; 61: 244–51.

345 Poskanzer DC, Walker AM, Prenney LB, Sheridan JL. The etiology of multiple sclerosis: temporal–spatial clustering indicating two environmental exposures before onset. Neurology 1981; 31: 708–13.

346 Cook SD, Blumberg B, Dowling PC, Deans W, Cross R. Multiple sclerosis and canine distemper on Key West, Florida. Lancet 1987; 1: 1426–7.

347 Benedikz J, Magnusson H, Guthmundsson G. Multiple sclerosis in Iceland, with observations on the alleged epidemic in the Faroe Islands. Ann Neurol 1994; 36(Suppl 2): S175–9.

348 Paul JR. Clinical Epidemiology, revised edition. Chicago: University of Chicago, 1966.

349 Tuohy VK, Yu M, Yin L et al. The epitope spreading cascade during progression of experimental autoimmune encephalomyelitis and multiple sclerosis. Immunol Rev 1998; 164: 93–100.

350 Comi G, Filippi M, Barkhof F et al. Effect of early interferon treatment on conversion to definite multiple sclerosis: a randomised study. Lancet 2001; 357: 1576–82.

351 Rabbins PV, Brooks BR, O'Donnell P et al. Structural brain correlates of emotional disorder in multiple sclerosis. Brain 1986; 109: 585–97.

352 Ron M, Feinstein A. Multiple sclerosis and the mind. J Neurol Neurosurg Psychiatry 1992; 545: 1–3.

353 Confavreux C, Compston DA, Hommes OR, McDonald WI, Thompson AJ. EDMUS, a European database for multiple sclerosis. J Neurol Neurosurg Psychiatry 1992; 55: 671–6.

354 Newton MR, Barrett G, Callanan MM, Towell AD. Cognitive event-related potentials in multiple sclerosis. Brain 1989; 112: 1637–60.

355 Pelosi L, Geesken JM, Holly M, Hayward M, Blumhardt LD. Working memory impairment in early multiple sclerosis. Evidence from an event-related potential study of patients with clinically isolated myelopathy. Brain 1997; 120: 2039–58.

356 Giesser BS, Schroeder MM, LaRocca NG et al. Endogenous event-related potentials as indices of dementia in multiple sclerosis patients. Electroencephalogr Clin Neurophysiol 1992; 82: 320–9.

357 Halliday AM, McDonald WI, Mushin J. Visual evoked response in diagnosis of multiple sclerosis. Br Med J 1973; 4: 661–4.

358 Ingram DA, Thompson AJ, Swash M. Central motor conduction in multiple sclerosis: evaluation of abnormalities revealed by transcutaneous magnetic stimulation of the brain. J Neurol Neurosurg Psychiatry 1988; 51: 487–94.

359 Celesia GG. Visual evoked potentials in clinical neurology. In: Aminof M, ed. Electrodiagnosis in Clinical Neurology. New York: Churchill-Livingstone, 1992: 467–89.

360 Comi G, Locatelli T, Leocani L. Confronto tra potenziali evocati somatosensoriali e test quantitativi delle sensibilità nei pazienti con sclerosi multipla. In: Comi G, ed. I Potenziali Evocati nella Sclerosi Multipla. Italy: Springer-Verlag, 1995: 85–90.

361 Comi G, Filippi M, Martinelli V et al. Brain stem magnetic resonance imaging and evoked potential studies of symptomatic multiple sclerosis patients. Eur Neurol 1993; 33: 232–7.

362 Nuwer MR, Packwood JW, Myers LW, Ellison GW. Evoked potentials predict the clinical changes in a multiple sclerosis drug study. Neurology 1987; 37: 1754–61.

363 La Mantia L, Riti F, Milanese C et al. Serial evoked potentials in multiple sclerosis bouts. Relation to steroid treatment. Ital J Neurol Sci 1994; 15: 333–40.

364 O'Connor P, Marchetti P, Lee L, Perera M. Evoked potential abnormality scores are a useful measure of disease burden in relapsing-remitting multiple sclerosis. Ann Neurol 1998; 44: 404–7.

365 Wingerchuk DM, Noseworthy JH, Weinshenker BG. Clinical outcome measures and rating scales in multiple sclerosis trials. Mayo Clin Proc 1997; 72: 1070–9.

366 Willoughby EW, Paty DW. Scales for rating impairment in multiple sclerosis: a critique. Neurology 1988; 38: 1793–8.

367 Hobart J, Freeman J, Thompson A. Kurtzke scales revisited: the application of psychometric methods to clinical intuition. Brain 2000; 123: 1027–40.

368 Goodkin DE, Cookfair D, Wende K et al. Inter- and intrarater scoring agreement using grades 1.0 to 3.5 of the Kurtzke Expanded Disability Status Scale (EDSS). Multiple Sclerosis Collaborative Research Group. Neurology 1992; 42: 859–63.

369 Noseworthy JH. Clinical scoring methods for multiple sclerosis. Ann Neurol 1994; 36: S80–5.

370 Goodkin DE, Hertsgaard D, Rudick RA. Exacerbation rates and adherence to disease type in a prospectively followed-up population with multiple sclerosis. Implications for clinical trials. Arch Neurol 1989; 46: 1107–12.

371 Rivers TM, Sprunt DH, Berry GP. Observations on attempts to produce acute disseminated encephalomyelitis in monkeys. J Exp Med 1933; 58: 39–53.

372 Martin R, McFarland HF, McFarlin DE. Immunological aspects of demyelinating diseases. Annu Rev Immunol 1992; 10: 153–87.

373 Constantinescu CS, Hilliard B, Fujioka T et al. Pathogenesis of neuroimmunologic diseases. Experimental models. Immunol Res 1998; 17: 217–27.

374 Ferraro A, Roizin L. Neuropathological variations in experimental allergic encephalomyelitis, hemorrhagic encephalomyelitis, perivenous encephalomyelitis, diffuse encephalomyelitis, patchy gliosis. J Neuropathol Exp Neurol 1954; 13: 60–89.

375 Sadovnick AD, Baird PA, Ward RH. Multiple sclerosis: updated risks for relatives. Am J Med Genet 1988; 29: 533–41.

376 Robertson NP, Clayton D, Fraser M, Deans J, Compston DA. Clinical concordance in sibling pairs with multiple sclerosis. Neurology 1996; 47: 347–52.

377 Mumford CJ, Wood NW, Kellar-Wood H et al. The British Isles survey of multiple sclerosis in twins. Neurology 1994; 44: 11–15.

378 Ebers GC, Sadovnick AD, Risch NJ. A genetic basis for familial aggregation in multiple sclerosis. Canadian Collaborative Study Group. Nature 1995; 377: 150–1.

379 Sadovnick AD, Ebers GC, Dyment DA, Risch NJ. Evidence for genetic basis of multiple sclerosis. The Canadian Collaborative Study Group. Lancet 1996; 347: 1728–30.

380 Rudick RA, Miller D, Clough JD, Gragg LA, Farmer RG. Quality of life in multiple sclerosis. Comparison with inflammatory bowel disease and rheumatoid arthritis. Arch Neurol 1992; 49: 1237–42.

381 Thorpe JW, Halpin SF, MacManus DG et al. A comparison between fast and conventional spin-echo in the detection of multiple sclerosis lesions. Neuroradiology 1994; 36: 388–92.

382 Rovaris M, Gawne-Cain ML, Wang L, Miller DH. A comparison of conventional and

fast spin-echo sequences for the measurement of lesion load in multiple sclerosis using a semi-automated contour technique. Neuroradiology 1997; 39: 161–5.

383 Krupp LB, Alvarez LA, LaRocca NG, Scheinberg LC. Fatigue in multiple sclerosis. Arch Neurol 1988; 45: 435–7.

384 Murray JT. Amantadine therapy for fatigue in multiple sclerosis. Can J Neurol Sci 1985; 12: 251–4.

385 van der Werf SP, Jongen PJH, Lycklama a Nijeholt GJ et al. Fatigue in multiple sclerosis: interrelations between fatigue complaints, cerebral MRI abnormalities and neurological disability. J Neurol Sci 1998; 160: 164–70.

386 Bakshi R. Miletich R., Henschel K et al. Fatigue in multiple sclerosis: cross-sectional correlation with brain MRI findings in 71 patients. Neurology 1999; 53: 1151–3.

387 Bakshi R, Shaikh ZA, Miletich RS et al. Fatigue in multiple sclerosis and its relationship to depression and neurologic disability. Mult Scler 2000; 6: 181–5.

388 Kroencke DC, Lynch SG, Denney DR. Fatigue in multiple sclerosis: relationship to depression, disability, and disease pattern. Mult Scler 2000; 6: 131–6.

389 Schwartz JE, Jandorf L, Krupp LB. The measurement of fatigue: a new instrument. J Psychosom Res 1993; 37: 753–62.

390 Fisk JD, Pontefract A, Ritvo PG, Archibald CJ, Murray TJ. The impact of fatigue on patients with multiple sclerosis. Can J Neurol Sci 1994; 21: 9–14.

391 Krupp LB, LaRocca NG, Muir-Nash J, Steinberg AD. The fatigue severity scale. Application to patients with multiple sclerosis and systemic lupus erythematosus. Arch Neurol 1989; 46: 1121–3.

392 Miller DH, Mac Manus DG et al. Detection of optic nerve lesions in optic neuritis using frequency-selective fat-saturation sequences. Neuroradiology 1993; 35: 156–8.

393 Fazekas F, Offenbacher H, Fuchs S et al. Criteria for an increased specificity of MRI interpretation in elderly subjects with suspected multiple sclerosis. Neurology 1988; 38: 1822–5.

394 Offenbacher H, Fazekas F, Schmidt R et al. Assessment of MRI criteria for a diagnosis of MS. Neurology 1993; 43: 905–9.

395 De Coene B, Hajnal JV, Gatehouse P et al. MR of the brain using fluid-attenuated inversion recovery (FLAIR) pulse sequences. AJNR 1992; 13: 1555–64.

396 Hendrix LE, Kneeland JB, Haughton VM et al. MR imaging of optic nerve lesions: value of gadopentetate dimeglumine and fat-suppression technique. AJNR 1990; 11: 749–54.

397 Cella DF, Dineen K, Arnason B et al. Validation of the functional assessment of multiple sclerosis quality of life instrument. Neurology 1996; 47: 129–39.

398 Hall KM, Hamilton BB, Waybe AG, Zasler MD. Characteristics and comparisons of functional assessment indices: Disability Rating Scale, Functional Independent Measure, and Functional Assessment Measure. J Head Trauma Rehabil 1993; 8: 60–74.

399 Kidd D, Stewart G, Baldry J et al. The Functional Independence Measure: a comparative validity and reliability study. Disabil Rehabil 1995; 17: 10–14.

400 Khan OA. Gabapentin relieves trigeminal neuralgia in multiple sclerosis patients. Neurology 1998; 51: 611–14.

401 Rosner H, Rubin L, Kestenbaum A. Gabapentin adjunctive therapy in neuropathic pain states. Clin J Pain 1996; 12: 56–8.

402 McFarland HF, Stone LA, Calabresi PA et al. MRI studies of multiple sclerosis: implications for the natural history of the disease and for monitoring effectiveness of experimental therapies. Mult Scler 1996; 2: 198–205.

403 Simon JH. Contrast-enhanced MR imaging in the evaluation of treatment response and prediction of outcome in multiple sclerosis. J Magn Reson Imaging 1997; 7: 29–37.

404 Kidd D, Thorpe JW, Kendall BE et al. MRI dynamics of brain and spinal cord in progressive multiple sclerosis. J Neurol Neurosurg Psychiatry 1996; 60: 15–19.

405 van Walderveen MA, Barkhof F, Hommes OR et al. Correlating MRI and clinical disease activity in multiple sclerosis: relevance of hypointense lesions on short-TR/short-TE (T1-weighted) spin-echo images. Neurology 1995; 45: 1684–90.

406 Kappos L, Moeri D, Radue EW et al. Predictive value of gadolinium-enhanced mag-netic resonance imaging for relapse rate and changes in disability or impairment in multiple sclerosis: a meta-analysis. Gadolinium MRI Meta-analysis Group. Lancet 1999; 353: 964–9.

407 Koudriavtseva T, Thompson AJ, Fiorelli M et al. Gadolinium enhanced MRI predicts clinical and MRI disease activity in relapsing-remitting multiple sclerosis. J Neurol Neurosurg Psychiatry 1997; 62: 285–7.

408 Molyneux PD, Filippi M, Barkhof F et al. Correlations between monthly enhanced MRI lesion rate and changes in T2 lesion volume in multiple sclerosis. Ann Neurol 1998; 43: 332–9.

409 Paty DW, Li DK. Interferon beta-1b is effective in relapsing-remitting multiple scler-osis. II. MRI analysis results of a multicenter, randomized, double-blind, placebo-controlled trial. UBC MS/MRI Study Group and the IFNB Multiple Sclerosis Study Group. Neurology 1993; 43: 662–7.

410 Miller DH, Molyneux PD, Barker GJ et al. Effect of interferon-beta1b on magnetic resonance imaging outcomes in secondary progressive multiple sclerosis: results of a European multicenter, randomized, double-blind, placebo-controlled trial. European Study Group on Interferon-beta1b in secondary progressive multiple sclerosis. Ann Neurol 1999; 46: 850–9.

411 Kurtzke JF, Beebe GW, Norman JEJ. Epidemiology of multiple sclerosis in US veter-ans. 1. Race, sex, and geographic distribution. Neurology 1979; 29: 1228–35.

412 Weinshenker BG, Santrach P, Bissonet AS et al. Major histocompatibility complex class II alleles and the course and outcome of MS: a population-based study. Neurology 1998; 51: 742–7.

413 McDonnell GV, Mawhinney H, Graham CA, Hawkins SA, Middleton D. A study of the HLA-DR region in clinical subgroups of multiple sclerosis and its influence. J Neurol Sci 1999; 165: 77–83.

414 Robertson NP, Fraser M, Deans J et al. Age-adjusted recurrence risks for relatives of patients with multiple sclerosis. Brain 1996; 119: 449–55.

415 Compston A. Genetic epidemiology of multiple sclerosis. J Neurol Neurosurg Psychiatry 1997; 62: 553–61.

416 Ben-Nun A, Mendel I, Bakimer R et al. The autoimmune reactivity to myelin oligo-dendrocyte glycoprotein (MOG) in multiple sclerosis is potentially pathogenic: effect of copolymer 1 on MOG-induced disease. J Neurol 1996; 243: S14–22.

417 Johnson KP, Brooks BR, Cohen JA et al. Extended use of glatiramer acetate (Copaxone) is well tolerated and maintains its clinical effect on multiple sclerosis relapse rate and degree of disability. Copolymer 1 Multiple Sclerosis Study Group. Neurology 1998; 50: 701–8.

418 Johnson KP, Brooks BR, Ford CC et al. Sustained clinical benefits of glatiramer acetate in relapsing multiple sclerosis patients observed for 6 years. Copolymer 1 Multiple Sclerosis Study Group. Mult Scler 2000; 6: 255–66.

419 Comi G, Filippi M, Wolinsky JS. European/Canadian multicenter, double-blind, ran-domized, placebo-controlled study of the effects of glatiramer acetate on magnetic resonance imaging – measured disease activity and burden in patients with relapsing multiple sclerosis. European/Canadian Glatiramer Acetate Study Group. Ann Neurol 2001; 49: 290–7.

420 Ge Y, Grossman RI, Udupa JK et al. Glatiramer acetate (Copaxone) treatment in relapsing-remitting MS: quantitative MR assessment. Neurology 2000; 54: 813–17.

421 Neuhaus O, Farina C, Wekerle H, Hohlfeld R. Mechanisms of action of glatiramer acetate in multiple sclerosis. Neurology 2001; 56: 702–8.

422 Ozawa K, Suchanek G, Breitschopf H et al. Patterns of oligodendroglia pathology in multiple sclerosis. Brain 1994; 117: 1311–22.

423 Mathewson AJ, Berry M. Observations on the astrocyte response to a cerebral stab wound in adult rats. Brain Res 1985; 327: 61–9.

424 Aisen ML, Holzer M, Rosen M, Dietz M, McDowell F. Glutethimide treatment of dis-abling action tremor in patients with multiple sclerosis and traumatic brain injury. Arch Neurol 1991; 48: 513–15.

425 Adams CW, Abdulla YH, Torres EM, Poston RN. Periventricular lesions in multiple sclerosis: their perivenous origin and relationship to granular ependymitis. Neuropathol Appl Neurobiol 1987; 13: 141–52.

426 Hoogervorst EL, van Winsen LM, Eikelenboom MJ et al. Comparisons of patient self-report, neurologic examination, and functional impairment in MS. Neurology 2001; 56: 934–7.

427 Schipper H, Clinch JJ, Olweny CLM. Quality of life studies: definitions and conceptural issues. In: Spilker B, ed. Quality of Life and Pharmacoeconomics in Clinical Trials. Philadelphia: Lippincott-Raven, 1996: 11–23.

428 Bergner M, Bobbitt RA, Carter WB, Gilson BS. The Sickness Impact Profile: development and final revision of a health status measure. Med Care 1981; 19: 787–805.

429 Hunt SM, McEwen J, McKenna SP. Measuring health status. London: Croom Helm, 1986.

430 Ware JE, Jr, Sherbourne CD. The MOS 36-item short-form health survey (SF-36). I. Conceptual framework and item selection. Med Care 1992; 30: 473–83.

431 Harding AE. The Hereditary Ataxia and Related Disorders. Edinburgh: Churchill Livingstone, 1984.

432 Haines JL, Ter-Minassian M, Bazyk A et al. A complete genomic screen for multiple sclerosis underscores a role for the major histocompatibility complex. The Multiple Sclerosis Genetics Group. Nat Genet 1996; 13: 469–71.

433 Sawcer S, Jones HB, Feakes R et al. A genome screen in multiple sclerosis reveals susceptibility loci on chromosome 6p21 and 17q22. Nat Genet 1996; 13: 464–8.

434 Compston A. Methods of genetic epidemiology in multiple sclerosis. In: Compston A, Ebers G, Lassmann H, McDonald I, Matthews B, Wekerle H, eds. McAlpine's Multiple Sclerosis. London: Churchill Livingstone, 1998: 45–61.

435 Guthrie TC. Visual and motor changes in patients with multiple sclerosis. A result of induced changes in environmental temperature. Arch Neurol Psychiatry 1951; 65: 437–51.

436 Guthrie TC, Nelson DA. Influence of temperature changes on multiple sclerosis: critical review of mechanisms and research potential. J Neurol Sci 1995; 129: 1–8.

437 Berger JR, Sheremata WA. Persistent neurological deficit precipitated by hot bath test in multiple sclerosis. JAMA 1983; 249: 1751–3.

438 Roman GC, Sheremata WA. Multiple sclerosis (not tropical spastic paraparesis) on Key West, Florida. Lancet 1987; 1: 1199.

439 Compston DA, Kellar Wood H, Robertson N, Sawcer S, Wood NW. Genes and susceptibility to multiple sclerosis. Acta Neurol Scand Suppl 1995; 161: 43–51.

440 Storch MK, Piddlesden S, Haltia M et al. Multiple sclerosis: in situ evidence for antibody- and complement-mediated demyelination. Ann Neurol 1998; 43: 465–71.

441 Reindl M, Linington C, Brehm U et al. Antibodies against the myelin oligodendrocyte glycoprotein and the myelin basic protein in multiple sclerosis and other neurological diseases: a comparative study. Brain 1999; 122: 2047–56.

442 Cross AH, Trotter JL, Lyons J. B cells and antibodies in CNS demyelinating disease. J Neuroimmunol 2001; 112: 1–14.

443 Sellebjerg F, Madsen HO, Frederiksen JL, Ryder LP, Svejgaard A. Acute optic neuritis: myelin basic protein and proteolipid protein antibodies, affinity, and the HLA system. Ann Neurol 1995; 38: 943–50.

444 Warren KG, Catz I. Relative frequency of autoantibodies to myelin basic protein and proteolipid protein in optic neuritis and multiple sclerosis cerebrospinal fluid. J Neurol Sci 1994; 121: 66–73.

445 Baig S, Olsson T, Yu-Ping J et al. Multiple sclerosis: cells secreting antibodies against myelin-associated glycoprotein are present in cerebrospinal fluid. Scand J Immunol 1991; 33: 73–9.

446 Lefvert AK, Link H. IgG production within the central nervous system: a critical review of proposed formulae. Ann Neurol 1985; 17: 13–20.

447 Huber SJ, Paulson GW, Shuttleworth EC et al. Magnetic resonance imaging correlates of dementia in multiple sclerosis. Arch Neurol 1987; 44: 732–6.

448 Fischer J. Using the Wechsler Memory Scale-Revised to detect and characterize memory deficits in multiple sclerosis. Clin Neuropsychol 1988; 2: 149–72.

449 Beatty WW. Memory and "frontal lobe" dysfunction in multiple sclerosis. J Neurol Sci 1993; 115(Suppl): S38–41.

450 Pandey JP, Goust JM, Salier JP, Fudenberg HH. Immunoglobulin G heavy chain (Gm) allotypes in multiple sclerosis. J Clin Invest 1981; 67: 1797–800.

451 Blanc M, Clanet M, Berr C et al. Immunoglobulin allotypes and susceptibility to multiple sclerosis. An epidemiological and genetic study in the Hautes-Pyrenees county of France. J Neurol Sci 1986; 75: 1–5.

452 Walter MA, Gibson WT, Ebers GC, Cox DW. Susceptibility to multiple sclerosis is associated with the proximal immunoglobulin heavy chain variable region. J Clin Invest 1991; 87: 1266–73.

453 Yu JS, Pandey JP, Massacesi L et al. Segregation of immunoglobulin heavy chain constant region genes in multiple sclerosis sibling pairs. J Neuroimmunol 1993; 42: 113–16

454 Hynes RO. Integrins: a family of cell surface receptors. Cell 1987; 48: 549–54.

455 Yednock TA, Cannon C, Fritz LC et al. Prevention of experimental autoimmune encephalomyelitis by antibodies against alpha 4 beta 1 integrin. Nature 1992; 356: 63–6.

456 Kraus J, Oschmann P, Engelhardt B et al. Soluble and cell surface ICAM-1 as markers for disease activity in multiple sclerosis. Acta Neurol Scand 1998; 98: 102–9.

457 Rieckmann P, Altenhofen B, Riegel A, Kallmann B, Felgenhauer K. Correlation of soluble adhesion molecules in blood and cerebrospinal fluid with magnetic resonance imaging activity in patients with multiple sclerosis. Mult Scler 1998; 4: 178–82.

458 Khoury SJ, Orav EJ, Guttmann CR et al. Changes in serum levels of ICAM and TNF–R correlate with disease activity in multiple sclerosis. Neurology 1999; 53: 758–64.

459 IFNB, Group TIMSSGatUoBCMMA. Interferon beta-1b in the treatment of multiple sclerosis. Neurology 1995; 45: 1277–85.

460 PRISMS. PRISMS-4: Long-term efficacy of interferon-beta-1a in relapsing MS. Neurology 2001; 56: 1628–36.

461 Panitch HS, Hirsch RL, Schindler J, Johnson KP. Treatment of multiple sclerosis with gamma interferon: exacerbations associated with activation of the immune system. Neurology 1987; 37: 1097–102.

462 De Maeyer E, De Maeyer-Guignard J. Induction of IFN-α and IFN-β. Interferons and Other Regulatory Cytokines. New York, NY: John Wiley & Sons Inc, 1988: 39–66.

463 Wandinger KP, Reissland P, Kirchner H, Wessel K, Otto M. Production of endogenous interferon-alpha and beta in patients with multiple sclerosis. J Neurol Neurosurg Psychiatry 1998; 64: 277–8.

464 Dettke M, Scheidt P, Prange H, Kirchner H. Correlation between interferon production and clinical disease activity in patients with multiple sclerosis. J Clin Immunol 1997; 17: 293–300.

465 Durelli L, Bongioanni MR, Ferrero B et al. Interferon alpha-2a treatment of relapsing-remitting multiple sclerosis: disease activity resumes after stopping treatment. Neurology 1996; 47: 123–9.

466 Squillacote D, Martinez M, Sheremata W. Natural alpha interferon in multiple sclerosis: results of three preliminary series. J Int Med Res 1996; 24: 246–57.

467 Blumhardt LD. Interferon beta-1a. In: Hawkins CP, Wolinsky JS, eds. Principles of Treatments in Multiple Sclerosis. Oxford: Butterworth Heinemann, 2000: 38–70.

468 Liberati AM, Garofani P, De Angelis V et al. Double-blind randomized phase I study on the clinical tolerance and pharmacodynamics of natural and recombinant interferon-beta given intravenously. J Interferon Res 1994; 14: 61–9.

469 IFNB. Neutralizing antibodies during treatment of multiple sclerosis with interferon beta-1b: experience during the first three years. The IFNB Multiple Sclerosis Study Group and the University of British Columbia MS/MRI Analysis Group. Neurology 1996; 47: 889–94.

470 Placebo-controlled multicentre randomised trial of interferon beta-1b in treatment

179

of secondary progressive multiple sclerosis. European Study Group on interferon beta-1b in secondary progressive MS. Lancet 1998; 352: 1491–7.

471 Goodkin DE. The North American study of interferon beta-1b in secondary progressive multiple sclerosis. American Academy of Neurology 52nd annual meeting, San Diego, USA, 2000.

472 Hohnoki K, Inoue A, Koh CS. Elevated serum levels of IFN-gamma, IL-4 and TNF-alpha/unelevated serum levels of IL-10 in patients with demyelinating diseases during the acute stage. J Neuroimmunol 1998; 87: 27–32.

473 Link J, Soderstrom M, Olsson T et al. Increased transforming growth factor-beta, interleukin-4, and interferon-gamma in multiple sclerosis. Ann Neurol 1994; 36: 379–86.

474 Vartanian T, Li Y, Zhao M, Stefansson K. Interferon-gamma-induced oligodendrocyte cell death: implications for the pathogenesis of multiple sclerosis. Mol Med 1995; 1: 732–43.

475 Vervliet G, Claeys H, Van Haver H et al. Interferon production and natural killer (NK) activity in leukocyte cultures from multiple sclerosis patients. J Neurol Sci 1983; 60: 137–50.

476 Brosnan CF, Cannella B, Battistini L, Raine CS. Cytokine localization in multiple sclerosis lesions: correlation with adhesion molecule expression and reactive nitrogen species. Neurology 1995; 45: S16–21.

477 Hauser SL, Doolittle TH, Lincoln R, Brown RH, Dinarello CA. Cytokine accumulations in CSF of multiple sclerosis patients: frequent detection of interleukin-1 and tumor necrosis factor but not interleukin-6. Neurology 1990; 40: 1735–9.

478 Cantrell DA, Smith KA. The interleukin-2 T-cell system: a new cell growth model. Science 1984; 224: 1312–16.

479 Trotter JL, Clifford DB, McInnis JE et al. Correlation of immunological studies and disease progression in chronic progressive multiple sclerosis. Ann Neurol 1989; 25: 172–8.

480 Freedman MS, Muth KL, Trotter JL, Yoshizawa CN, Antel JP. Prospective serial analysis of interleukin-2 and soluble interleukin-2 receptor in relapsing-remitting multiple sclerosis. Neurology 1992; 42: 1596–601.

481 Trotter JL, Damico CA, Trotter AL, Collins KG, Cross AH. Interleukin-2 binding proteins in sera from normal subjects and multiple sclerosis patients. Neurology 1995; 45: 1971–4.

482 Hofman FM, von Hanwehr RI, Dinarello CA et al. Immunoregulatory molecules and IL 2 receptors identified in multiple sclerosis brain. J Immunol 1986; 136: 3239–45.

483 Hartung HP, Hughes RA, Taylor WA et al. T cell activation in Guillain-Barre syndrome and in MS: elevated serum levels of soluble IL-2 receptors. Neurology 1990; 40: 215–18.

484 Bansil S, Troiano R, Cook SD, Rohowsky-Kochan C. Serum soluble interleukin-2 receptor levels in chronic progressive, stable and steroid-treated multiple sclerosis. Acta Neurol Scand 1991; 84: 282–5.

485 Sharief MK, Thompson EJ. Correlation of interleukin-2 and soluble interleukin-2 receptor with clinical activity of multiple sclerosis. J Neurol Neurosurg Psychiatry 1993; 56: 169–74.

486 Kittur SD, Kittur DS, Soncrant TT et al. Soluble interleukin-2 receptors in cerebrospinal fluid from individuals with various neurological disorders. Ann Neurol 1990; 28: 168–73.

487 Gallo P, Piccinno MG, Tavolato B, Siden A. A longitudinal study on IL-2, sIL-2R, IL-4 and IFN-gamma in multiple sclerosis CSF and serum. J Neurol Sci 1991; 101: 227–32.

488 Navikas V, Link H. Review: cytokines and the pathogenesis of multiple sclerosis. J Neurosci Res 1996; 45: 322–33.

489 Gausling R, Trollmo C, Hafler DA. Decreases in interleukin-4 secretion by invariant CD4(-)CD8(-)V alpha 24J alpha Q T cells in peripheral blood of patients with relapsing-remitting multiple sclerosis. Clin Immunol 2001; 98: 11–17.

490 Soderstrom M, Hillert J, Link J et al. Expression of IFN-gamma, IL-4, and TGF-beta in

multiple sclerosis in relation to HLA-Dw2 phenotype and stage of disease. Mult Scler 1995; 1: 173–80.

491   Vercelli D, Jabara HH, Lauener RP, Geha RS. IL-4 inhibits the synthesis of IFN-gamma and induces the synthesis of IgE in human mixed lymphocyte cultures. J Immunol 1990; 144: 570–3.

492   Howard M, O'Garra A, Ishida H et al. Biological properties of interleukin 10. J Clin Immunol 1992; 12: 239–47.

493   Rieckmann P, Albrecht M, Kitze B et al. Tumor necrosis factor-alpha messenger RNA expression in patients with relapsing-remitting multiple sclerosis is associated with disease activity. Ann Neurol 1995; 37: 82–8.

494   Salmaggi A, Dufour A, Eoli M et al. Low serum interleukin-10 levels in multiple sclerosis: further evidence for decreased systemic immunosuppression? J Neurol 1996; 243: 13–17.

495   Ozenci V, Kouwenhoven M, Huang YM et al. Multiple sclerosis: levels of interleukin-10-secreting blood mononuclear cells are low in untreated patients but augmented during interferon-beta-1b treatment. Scand J Immunol 1999; 49: 554–61.

496   van Boxel-Dezaire AH, Hoff SC, van Oosten BW et al. Decreased interleukin-10 and increased interleukin-12p40 mRNA are associated with disease activity and characterize different disease stages in multiple sclerosis. Ann Neurol 1999; 45: 695–703.

497   Rudick RA, Ransohoff RM, Lee JC et al. In vivo effects of interferon beta-1a on immunosuppressive cytokines in multiple sclerosis. Neurology 1998; 50: 1294–300.

498   Rep MH, Schrijver HM, van Lopik T et al. Interferon (IFN)-beta treatment enhances CD95 and interleukin 10 expression but reduces interferon-gamma producing T cells in MS patients. J Neuroimmunol 1999; 96: 92–100.

499   Smith JL, Cogan DG. Internuclear ophthalmoplegia: a review of fifty-eight cases. Arch Ophthalmol 1959; 61: 687–95.

500   Atlas SW, Grossman RI, Savino PJ et al. Interunclear ophthalmoplegia: MR-anatomic correlation. AJNR 1987; 8: 243–7.

501   Prineas JW, Wright RG. Macrophages, lymphocytes, and plasma cells in the perivascular compartment in chronic multiple sclerosis. Lab Invest 1978; 38: 409–21.

502   Simpson JF, Tourtellotte WW, Kokmen E, Parker JA, Itabashi HH. Fluorescent protein tracing in multiple sclerosis brain tissue. Arch Neurol 1969; 20: 373–7.

503   Fazekas F, Deisenhammer F, Strasser-Fuchs S, Nahler G, Mamoli B. Randomised placebo-controlled trial of monthly intravenous immunoglobulin therapy in relapsing-remitting multiple sclerosis. Austrian Immunoglobulin in Multiple Sclerosis Study Group. Lancet 1997; 349: 589–93.

504   Fazekas F, Deisenhammer F, Strasser-Fuchs S, Nahler G, Mamoli B. Treatment effects of monthly intravenous immunoglobulin on patients with relapsing-remitting multiple sclerosis: further analyses of the Austrian Immunoglobulin in MS study. Mult Scler 1997; 3: 137–41.

505   Sorensen PS, Wanscher B, Jensen CV et al. Intravenous immunoglobulin G reduces MRI activity in relapsing multiple sclerosis. Neurology 1998; 50: 1273–81.

506   Orvieto R, Achiron R, Rotstein Z et al. Pregnancy and multiple sclerosis: a 2-year experience. Eur J Obstet Gynecol Reprod Biol 1999; 82: 191–4.

507   Fazekas F, Gold R, Hartung HP, Strasser-Fuchs S. Immunoglobulins. In: Hawkins CP, Wolinsky JS, eds. Principles of Treatments in Multiple Sclerosis. Oxford: Butterworth Heinemann, 2000: 95–113.

508   Francis DA, Grundy D, Heron JR. The response to isoniazid of action tremor in multiple sclerosis and its assessment using polarised light goniometry. J Neurol Neurosurg Psychiatry 1986; 49: 87–9.

509   Bozek CB, Kastrukoff LF, Wright JM, Perry TL, Larsen TA. A controlled trial of isoniazid therapy for action tremor in multiple sclerosis. J Neurol 1987; 234: 36–9.

510   Milligan NM, Miller DH, Compston DA. A placebo-controlled trial of isoprinosine in patients with multiple sclerosis. J Neurol Neurosurg Psychiatry 1994; 57: 164–8.

511   Harding AE, Sweeney MG, Miller DH et al. Occurrence of a multiple sclerosis-like illness in women who have a Leber's hereditary optic neuropathy mitochondrial DNA mutation. Brain 1992; 115: 979–89.

512 Howell N, Kubacka I, Xu M, McCullough DA. Leber hereditary optic neuropathy: involvement of the mitochondrial ND1 gene and evidence for an intragenic suppressor mutation. Am J Hum Genet 1991; 48: 935–42.

513 Huoponen K, Vilkki J, Aula P, Nikoskelainen EK, Savontaus ML. A new mtDNA mutation associated with Leber hereditary optic neuroretinopathy. Am J Hum Genet 1991; 48: 1147–53.

514 Baker D, Butler D, Scallon BJ et al. Control of established experimental allergic encephalomyelitis by inhibition of tumor necrosis factor (TNF) activity within the central nervous system using monoclonal antibodies and TNF receptor-immunoglobulin fusion proteins. Eur J Immunol 1994; 24: 2040–8.

515 Klinkert WE, Kojima K, Lesslauer W et al. TNF-alpha receptor fusion protein prevents experimental auto-immune encephalomyelitis and demyelination in Lewis rats: an overview. J Neuroimmunol 1997; 72: 163–8.

516 Lenercept, Group MSS. TNF neutralization in MS: results of a randomized, placebo-controlled multicenter study. The Lenercept Multiple Sclerosis Study Group and The University of British Columbia MS/MRI Analysis Group. Neurology 1999; 53: 457–65.

517 Lassmann H. Neuropathology in multiple sclerosis: new concepts. Mult Scler 1998; 4: 93–8.

518 Eldridge R, Anayiotos CP, Schlesinger S et al. Hereditary adult-onset leukodystrophy simulating chronic progressive multiple sclerosis. N Engl J Med 1984; 311: 948–53.

519 Samuelsson B, Dahlen SE, Lindgren JA, Rouzer CA, Serhan CN. Leukotrienes and lipoxins: structures, biosynthesis, and biological effects. Science 1987; 237: 1171–6.

520 Neu I, Mallinger J, Wildfeuer A, Mehlber L. Leukotrienes in the cerebrospinal fluid of multiple sclerosis patients. Acta Neurol Scand 1992; 86: 586–7.

521 Rosnowska M, Cendrowski W, Sobczyk W. [Leukotrienes B4 and C4 in cerebrospinal of patients with multiple sclerosis]. Pol Merkuriusz Lek 1997; 2: 254–5.

522 Massaro AR, Cioffi RP, Laudisio A, Schiavino D, Mariani M. Four year double-blind controlled study of levamisole in multiple sclerosis. Ital J Neurol Sci 1990; 11: 595–9.

523 Cendrowski W, Czlonkowska A. Levamisole in multiple sclerosis; with special reference to immunological parameters. A pilot study. Acta Neurol Scand 1978; 57: 354–9.

524 Gonsette RE, Demonty L, Delmotte P et al. Modulation of immunity in multiple sclerosis: a double-blind levamisole-placebo controlled study in 85 patients. J Neurol 1982; 228: 65–72.

525 Lhermitte J, Bollak J, Nicolas M. Les douleurs a type de decharge electrique consecutives a la flexion cephalique dans la sclerose en plaques: un cas de forme sensitive de la sclerose multiple. Revue Neurol 1924; 31: 56–62.

526 Kanchandani R, Howe JG. Lhermitte's sign in multiple sclerosis: a clinical survey and review of the literature. J Neurol Neurosurg Psychiatry 1982; 45: 308–12.

527 Gutrecht JA, Zamani AA, Salgado ED. Anatomic-radiologic basis of Lhermitte's sign in multiple sclerosis. Arch Neurol 1993; 50: 849–52.

528 Fogdell A, Olerup O, Fredrikson S, Vrethem M, Hillert J. Linkage analysis of HLA class II genes in Swedish multiplex families with multiple sclerosis. Neurology 1997; 48: 758–62.

529 Harwood RH, Rogers A, Dickinson E, Ebrahim S. Measuring handicap: the London Handicap Scale, a new outcome measure for chronic disease. Qual Health Care 1994; 3: 11–16.

530 Thompson AJ. Measuring handicap in multiple sclerosis. Mult Scler 1999; 5: 260–2.

531 Tulving E. Episodic and semantic memory In: Organization of memory. Tulving E, Donaldson W, eds. New York: Academic Press, 1972.

532 Coyle PK. Borrelia burgdorferi antibodies in multiple sclerosis patients. Neurology 1989; 39: 760–1.

533 Lieberman AP, Pitha PM, Shin HS, Shin ML. Production of tumor necrosis factor and other cytokines by astrocytes stimulated with lipopolysaccharide or a neurotropic virus. Proc Natl Acad Sci USA 1989; 86: 6348–52.

534 Cannella B, Raine CS. The adhesion molecule and cytokine profile of multiple sclerosis lesions. Ann Neurol 1995; 37: 424–35.

535 Navikas V, He B, Link J, Haglund M et al. Augmented expression of tumour necrosis factor-alpha and lymphotoxin in mononuclear cells in multiple sclerosis and optic neuritis. Brain 1996; 119: 213–23.

536 Selmaj K, Raine CS, Cross AH. Anti-tumor necrosis factor therapy abrogates autoimmune demyelination. Ann Neurol 1991; 30: 694–700.

537 Arnold DL, Wolinsky JS, Matthews PM, Falini A. The use of magnetic resonance spectroscopy in the evaluation of the natural history of multiple sclerosis. J Neurol Neurosurg Psychiatry 1998; 64(Suppl 1): S94–101.

538 Bjartmar C, Kidd G, Mork S, Rudick R, Trapp BD. Neurological disability correlates with spinal cord axonal loss and reduced N-acetyl aspartate in chronic multiple sclerosis patients. Ann Neurol 2000; 48: 893–901.

539 Brant–Zawadzki M, Gillan GD, Nitz WR. MP RAGE: a three-dimensional, T1-weighted, gradient-echo sequence – initial experience in the brain. Radiology 1992; 182: 769–75.

540 Filippi M, Yousry T, Horsfield MA et al. A high-resolution three-dimensional T1-weighted gradient echo sequence improves the detection of disease activity in multiple sclerosis. Ann Neurol 1996; 40: 901–7.

541 Filippi M, Rocca MA, Horsfield MA et al. Increased spatial resolution using a three-dimensional T1-weighted gradient-echo MR sequence results in greater hypointense lesion volumes in multiple sclerosis. Am J Neuroradiol 1998; 19: 235-8.

542 Wolff SD, Balaban RS. Magnetization transfer imaging: practical aspects and clinical applications. Radiology 1994; 192: 593–9.

543 Filippi M, Campi A, Mammi S et al. Brain magnetic resonance imaging and multimodal evoked potentials in benign and secondary progressive multiple sclerosis. J Neurol Neurosurg Psychiatry 1995; 58: 31–7.

544 Phillips MD, Grossman RI, Miki Y et al. Comparison of T2 lesion volume and magnetization transfer ratio histogram analysis and of atrophy and measures of lesion burden in patients with multiple sclerosis. AJNR 1998; 19: 1055–60.

545 Richert ND, Frank JA. Magnetization transfer imaging to monitor clinical trials in multiple sclerosis. Neurology 1999; 53: S29–32.

546 van Buchem MA, Grossman RI, Armstrong C et al. Correlation of volumetric magnetization transfer imaging with clinical data in MS. Neurology 1998; 50: 1609–17.

547 Rovaris M, Filippi M, Falautano M et al. Relation between MR abnormalities and patterns of cognitive impairment in multiple sclerosis. Neurology 1998; 50: 1601–8.

548 Currier RD, Haerer AF, Meydrech EF. Low dose oral methotrexate treatment of multiple sclerosis: a pilot study. J Neurol Neurosurg Psychiatry 1993; 56: 1217–18.

549 Goodkin DE, Rudick RA, VanderBrug Medendorp S et al. Low-dose (7.5 mg) oral methotrexate reduces the rate of progression in chronic progressive multiple sclerosis. Ann Neurol 1995; 37: 30–40.

550 Fischer JS, Goodkin DE, Rudick RA. Low-dose (7.5 mg) oral methotrexate improves neuropsychological function in patients with chronic progressive multiple sclerosis. Double-blind crossover and three-year study. Ann Neurol 1994; 36: 289.

551 Goodkin DE, Rudick RA, VanderBrug Medendorp S, Daughtry MM, Van Dyke C. Low-dose oral methotrexate in chronic progressive multiple sclerosis: analyses of serial MRIs. Neurology 1996; 47: 1153–7.

552 Detels R, Visscher BR, Hayle RW et al. Evidence for lower susceptibility to multiple sclerosis in Japanese-Americans. Am J Epidemiol 1978; 108: 386–93.

553 Weinshenker BG, Bass B, Rice GP et al. The natural history of multiple sclerosis: a geographically based study. 2. Predictive value of an early clinical course. Brain 1989; 112: 1419–28.

554 Reder AT, Arnason BG. Trigeminal neuralgia in multiple sclerosis relieved by a prostaglandin E analogue. Neurology 1995; 45: 1097–100.

555 Attardi G, Schatz G. Biogenesis of mitochondria. Annu Rev Cell Biol 1988; 4: 289–333.

556 Riordan-Eva P, Sanders MD, Govan GG et al. The clinical features of Leber's heredi-

tary optic neuropathy defined by the presence of a pathogenic mitochondrial DNA mutation. Brain 1995; 118: 319–37.

557 Hogancamp WE, Rodriguez M, Weinshenker BG. Identification of multiple sclerosis-associated genes. Mayo Clin Proc 1997; 72: 965–76.

558 Krapf H, Mauch E, Fetzer U, Laufen H, Kornhuber HH. Serial gadolinium-enhanced magnetic resonance imaging in patients with multiple sclerosis treated with mitoxantrone. Neuroradiology 1995; 37: 113–19.

559 Edan G, Miller D, Clanet M et al. Therapeutic effect of mitoxantrone combined with methylprednisolone in multiple sclerosis: a randomised multicentre study of active disease using MRI and clinical criteria. J Neurol Neurosurg Psychiatry 1997; 62: 112–18.

560 Krapf H, Morrissey S, Zenker O. Mitoxantrone in progressive multiple sclerosis: a placebo-controlled, randomized, oberver-blind European phase III study. MRI data. Mult Scler 1998; 4: 380.

561 Hartung HP, Gonsette R, Konig N et al. Mitoxantrone in progressive multiple sclerosis: a placebo-controlled, double-blind, randomised, multicentre trial. Lancet 2002; 360: 2018–25.

562 Edan G, Morrisey S. Mitoxantrone. In: Hawkins CP, Wolinsky JS, eds. Principles of Treatments in Multiple Sclerosis. Oxford: Butterworth Heinemann, 2000: 131–46.

563 Millefiorini E, Gasperini C, Pozzilli C, D'Andrea F, Bastianello S, Trojano M, et al. Randomized placebo-controlled trial of mitoxantrone in relapsing-remitting multiple sclerosis: 24-month clinical and MRI outcome. J Neurol 1997; 244: 153–9.

564 Merton PA, Morton HB. Stimulation of the cerebral cortex in the intact human subject. Nature 1980; 285: 227.

565 Cowan JM, Rothwell JC, Dick JP, Thompson PD, Day BL, Marsden CD. Abnormalities in central motor pathway conduction in multiple sclerosis. Lancet 1984; 2: 304–7.

566 Paty DW, Oger JJ, Kastrukoff LF et al. MRI in the diagnosis of MS: a prospective study with comparison of clinical evaluation, evoked potentials, oligoclonal banding, and CT. Neurology 1988; 38: 180–5.

567 Miller DH, Grossman RI, Reingold SC, McFarland HF. The role of magnetic resonance techniques in understanding and managing multiple sclerosis. Brain 1998; 121: 3–24.

568 Tas MW, Barkhol F, van Walderveen MA et al. The effect of gadolinium on the sensitivity and specificity of MR in the initial diagnosis of multiple sclerosis. AJNR 1995; 16: 259–64.

569 Rice G, Ebers G. Interferons in the treatment of multiple sclerosis: do they prevent the progression of the disease? Arch Neurol 1998; 55: 1578–80.

570 Simon JH, Jacobs LD, Campion M et al. Magnetic resonance studies of intramuscular interferon beta-1a for relapsing multiple sclerosis. The Multiple Sclerosis Collaborative Research Group. Ann Neurol 1998; 43: 79–87.

571 Rudick RA, Fisher E, Lee JC, Simon J, Jacobs L. Use of the brain parenchymal fraction to measure whole brain atrophy in relapsing-remitting MS. Multiple Sclerosis Collaborative Research Group. Neurology 1999; 53: 1698–704.

572 Schwid SR, Goodman AD, Mattson DH et al. The measurement of ambulatory impairment in multiple sclerosis. Neurology 1997; 49: 1419–24.

573 Fischer JS, Rudick RA, Cutter GR, Reingold SC. The Multiple Sclerosis Functional Composite Measure (MSFC): an integrated approach to MS clinical outcome assessment. National MS Society Clinical Outcomes Assessment Task Force. Mult Scler 1999; 5: 244–50.

574 Cohen JA, Fischer JS, Bolibrush DM et al. Intrarater and interrater reliability of the MS functional composite outcome measure. Neurology 2000; 54: 802–6.

575 Kalkers NF, de Groot V, Lazeron RH et al. MS functional composite: relation to disease phenotype and disability strata. Neurology 2000; 54: 1233–9.

576 Kalkers NF, Bergers L, de Groot V et al. Concurrent validity of the MS Functional Composite using MRI as a biological disease marker. Neurology 2001; 56: 215–19.

577 Miller DM, Rudick RA, Cutter G, Baier M, Fischer JS. Clinical significance of the mul-

tiple sclerosis functional composite: relationship to patient-reported quality of life. Arch Neurol 2000; 57: 1319–24.

578 Rudick RA, Cutter G, Baier M et al. Use of the Multiple Sclerosis Functional Composite to predict disability in relapsing MS. Neurology 2001; 56: 1324–30.

579 Hoogervorst EL, Kalkers NF, Uitdehaag BM, Polman CH. A study validating changes in the multiple sclerosis functional composite. Arch Neurol 2002; 59: 113–16.

580 Fischer JS, Jack AJ, Knicker JE. Administration and Scoring Manual for the Multiple Sclerosis Functional Composite Measure (MSFC). New York, NY: Demos Medical Publishing Inc, 1999.

581 Vickrey BG, Hays RD, Harooni R, Myers LW, Ellison GW. A health-related quality of life measure for multiple sclerosis. Qual Life Res 1995; 4: 187–206.

582 Janardhan V, Bakshi R. Quality of life and its relationship to brain lesions and atrophy on magnetic resonance images in 60 patients with multiple sclerosis. Arch Neurol 2000; 57: 1485–91.

583 Fischer JS, LaRocca NG, Miller DM et al. Recent developments in the assessment of quality of life in multiple sclerosis (MS). Mult Scler 1999; 5: 251–9.

584 Giesser BS, Kurtzberg D, Vaughan HG et al. Trimodal evoked potentials compared with magnetic resonance imaging in the diagnosis of multiple sclerosis. Arch Neurol 1987; 44: 281–4.

585 Gilmore RL, Kasarskis EJ, Carr WA, Norvell E. Comparative impact of paraclinical studies in establishing the diagnosis of multiple sclerosis. Electroencephalogr Clin Neurophysiol 1989; 73: 433–42.

586 Hume AL, Waxman SG. Evoked potentials in suspected multiple sclerosis: diagnostic value and prediction of clinical course. J Neurol Sci 1988; 83: 191–210.

587 Nyenhuis DL, Rao SM, Zajecka JM et al. Mood disturbance versus other symptoms of depression in multiple sclerosis. J Int Neuropsychol Soc 1995; 1: 291–6.

588 Ritchie JM. Myelin. In: Morell P, ed. Myelin. New York: Plenum, 1984: 117–46.

589 Schmidt S. Candidate autoantigens in multiple sclerosis. Mult Scler 1999; 5: 147–60.

590 Berger T, Weerth S, Kojima K et al. Experimental autoimmune encephalomyelitis: the antigen specificity of T lymphocytes determines the topography of lesions in the central and peripheral nervous system. Lab Invest 1997; 76: 355–64.

591 Weerth S, Berger T, Lassmann H, Linington C. Encephalitogenic and neuritogenic T cell responses to the myelin-associated glycoprotein (MAG) in the Lewis rat. J Neuroimmunol 1999; 95: 157–64.

592 Zhang Y, Burger D, Saruhan G, Jeannet M, Steck AJ. The T-lymphocyte response against myelin-associated glycoprotein and myelin basic protein in patients with multiple sclerosis. Neurology 1993; 43: 403–7.

593 Cohen SR, Brooks BR, Herndon RM, McKhann GM. A diagnostic index of active demyelination: myelin basic protein in cerebrospinal fluid. Ann Neurol 1980; 8: 25–31.

594 Lamers KJ, de Reus HP, Jongen PJ. Myelin basic protein in CSF as indicator of disease activity in multiple sclerosis. Mult Scler 1998; 4: 124–6.

595 Sellebjerg F, Christiansen M, Nielsen PM, Frederiksen JL. Cerebrospinal fluid measures of disease activity in patients with multiple sclerosis. Mult Scler 1998; 4: 475–9.

596 Mithen FA, Agrawal HC, Eylar EH et al. Studies with antisera against peripheral nervous system myelin and myelin basic proteins. I. Effects of antiserum upon living cultures of nervous tissue. Brain Res 1982; 250: 321–31.

597 Mithen FA, Agrawal HC, Fishman MA, Eylar EH, Bunge RP. Studies with antisera against peripheral nervous system myelin and myelin basic proteins. II. Immunohistochemical studies in cultures of rat dorsal root ganglion neurons and Schwann cells. Brain Res 1982; 250: 333–43.

598 Kerlero de Rosbo N, Milo R, Lees MB et al. Reactivity to myelin antigens in multiple sclerosis. Peripheral blood lymphocytes respond predominantly to myelin oligodendrocyte glycoprotein. J Clin Invest 1993; 92: 2602–8.

599 Kerlero de Rosbo N, Hoffman M, Mendel I et al. Predominance of the autoimmune response to myelin oligodendrocyte glycoprotein (MOG) in multiple sclerosis:

reactivity to the extracellular domain of MOG is directed against three main regions. Eur J Immunol 1997; 27: 3059–69.

600 Tienari PJ, Terwilliger JD, Ott J, Palo J, Peltonen L. Two-locus linkage analysis in multiple sclerosis (MS). Genomics 1994; 19: 320–5.

601 He B, Yang B, Lundahl J, Fredrikson S, Hillert J. The myelin basic protein gene in multiple sclerosis: identification of discrete alleles of a 1.3 kb tetranucleotide repeat sequence. Acta Neurol Scand 1998; 97: 46–51.

602 Eoli M, Pandolfo M, Milanese C et al. The myelin basic protein gene is not a major susceptibility locus for multiple sclerosis in Italian patients. J Neurol 1994; 241: 615–19.

603 Cohen SR, Herndon RM, McKhann GM. Myelin basic protein in cerebrospinal fluid as an indicator of active demyelination. Trans Am Neurol Assoc 1976; 101: 45–7.

604 Whitaker JN. Myelin basic protein in cerebrospinal fluid and other body fluids. Mult Scler 1998; 4: 16–21.

605 Whitaker JN, Kachelhofer RD, Bradley EL et al. Urinary myelin basic protein-like material as a correlate of the progression of multiple sclerosis. Ann Neurol 1995; 38: 625–32.

606 Whitaker JN, Layton BA, Bartolucci AA et al. Urinary myelin basic protein-like material in patients with multiple sclerosis during interferon beta-1b treatment. Arch Neurol 1999; 56: 687–91.

607 Linington C, Bradl M, Lassmann H, Brunner C, Vass K. Augmentation of demyelination in rat acute allergic encephalomyelitis by circulating mouse monoclonal antibodies directed against a myelin/oligodendrocyte glycoprotein. Am J Pathol 1988; 130: 443–54.

608 Adelmann M, Wood J, Benzel I et al. The N–terminal domain of the myelin oligodendrocyte glycoprotein (MOG) induces acute demyelinating experimental autoimmune encephalomyelitis in the Lewis rat. J Neuroimmunol 1995; 63: 17–27.

609 Genain CP, Nguyen MH, Letvin NL et al. Antibody facilitation of multiple sclerosis-like lesions in a nonhuman primate. J Clin Invest 1995; 96: 2966–74.

610 Kaye JF, Kerlero de Rosbo N, Mendel I et al. The central nervous system-specific myelin oligodendrocytic basic protein (MOBP) is encephalitogenic and a potential target antigen in multiple sclerosis (MS). J Neuroimmunol 2000; 102: 189–98.

611 Storch MK, Stefferl A, Brehm U et al. Autoimmunity to myelin oligodendrocyte glycoprotein in rats mimics the spectrum of multiple sclerosis pathology. Brain Pathol 1998; 8: 681–94.

612 Mithen F, Bunge R, Agrawal H. Proteolipid protein antiserum does not affect CNS myelin in rat spinal cord culture. Brain Res 1980; 197: 477–83.

613 Seil FJ, Agrawal HC. Myelin-proteolipid protein does not induce demyelinating or myelination-inhibiting antibodies. Brain Res 1980; 194: 273–7.

614 Constantinescu CS, Wysocka M, Hilliard B et al. Antibodies against IL-12 prevent superantigen-induced and spontaneous relapses of experimental autoimmune encephalomyelitis. J Immunol 1998; 161: 5097–104.

615 Nakano M, Ueda H, Li JY, Matsumoto M, Yanagihara T. Measurement of regional N-acetylaspartate after transient global ischemia in gerbils with and without ischemic tolerance: an index of neuronal survival. Ann Neurol 1998; 44: 334–40.

616 Huber C, Batchelor JR, Fuchs D et al. Immune response-associated production of neopterin. Release from macrophages primarily under control of interferon-gamma. J Exp Med 1984; 160: 310–16.

617 Ott M, Demisch L, Engelhardt W, Fischer PA. Interleukin-2, soluble interleukin-2-receptor, neopterin, L-tryptophan and beta 2-microglobulin levels in CSF and serum of patients with relapsing-remitting or chronic-progressive multiple sclerosis. J Neurol 1993; 241: 108–14.

618 Shaw CE, Dunbar PR, Macaulay HA, Neale TJ. Measurement of immune markers in the serum and cerebrospinal fluid of multiple sclerosis patients during clinical remission. J Neurol 1995; 242: 53–8.

619 Giovannoni G, Lai M, Kidd D et al. Daily urinary neopterin excretion as an

immunological marker of disease activity in multiple sclerosis. Brain 1997; 120: 1–13.

620 Lycke JN, Karlsson J-E, Andersen O, Rosengren LE. Neurofilament protein in cerebrospinal fluid: a potential marker of activity in multiple sclerosis. J Neurol Neurosurg Psychiatry 1997; 64: 401–4.

621 Moncada S, Higgs A. The L-arginine-nitric oxide pathway. N Engl J Med 1993; 329: 2002–12.

622 Merrill JE, Ignarro LJ, Sherman MP, Melinek J, Lane TE. Microglial cell cytotoxicity of oligodendrocytes is mediated through nitric oxide. J Immunol 1993; 151: 2132–41.

623 Oleszak EL, Zaczynska E, Bhattacharjee M et al. Inducible nitric oxide synthase and nitrotyrosine are found in monocytes/macrophages and/or astrocytes in acute, but not in chronic, multiple sclerosis. Clin Diagn Lab Immunol 1998; 5: 438–45.

624 Johnson AW, Land JM, Thompson EJ et al. Evidence for increased nitric oxide production in multiple sclerosis. J Neurol Neurosurg Psychiatry 1995; 58: 107.

625 Giovannoni G, Heales SJ, Land JM, Thompson EJ. The potential role of nitric oxide in multiple sclerosis. Mult Scler 1998; 4: 212–16.

626 Bo L, Dawson TM, Wesselingh S et al. Induction of nitric oxide synthase in demyelinating regions of multiple sclerosis brains. Ann Neurol 1994; 36: 778–86.

627 Allen IV, McKeown SR. A histological, histochemical and biochemical study of the macroscopically normal white matter in multiple sclerosis. J Neurol Sci 1979; 41: 81–91.

628 Barbosa S, Blumhardt LD, Roberts N, Lock T, Edwards RH. Magnetic resonance relaxation time mapping in multiple sclerosis: normal appearing white matter and the "invisible" lesion load. Magn Reson Imaging 1994; 12: 33–42.

629 Filippi M, Campi A, Dousset V et al. A magnetization transfer imaging study of normal-appearing white matter in multiple sclerosis. Neurology 1995; 45: 478–82.

630 Tortorella C, Viti B, Bozzali M et al. A magnetization transfer histogram study of normal-appearing brain tissue in MS. Neurology 2000; 54: 186–93.

631 Filippi M, Rocca MA, Martino G, Horsfield MA, Comi G. Magnetization transfer changes in the normal appearing white matter precede the appearance of enhancing lesions in patients with multiple sclerosis. Ann Neurol 1998; 43: 809–14.

632 Filippi M, Tortorella C, Bozzali M. Normal-appearing white matter changes in multiple sclerosis: the contribution of magnetic resonance techniques. Mult Scler 1999; 5: 273–82.

633 McLean BN, Luxton RW, Thompson EJ. A study of immunoglobulin G in the cerebrospinal fluid of 1007 patients with suspected neurological disease using isoelectric focusing and the Log IgG-Index. A comparison and diagnostic applications. Brain 1990; 113: 1269–89.

634 Raine CS. The Norton Lecture: a review of the oligodendrocyte in the multiple sclerosis lesion. J Neuroimmunol 1997; 77: 135–52.

635 Bruck W, Schmied M, Suchanek G et al. Oligodendrocytes in the early course of multiple sclerosis. Ann Neurol 1994; 35: 65–73.

636 Raine CS, Wu E. Multiple sclerosis: remyelination in acute lesions. J Neuropathol Exp Neurol 1993; 52: 199–204.

637 Sharief MK. Cytokines in multiple sclerosis: pro-inflammation or pro-remyelination? Mult Scler 1998; 4: 169–73.

638 Dowling P, Ming X, Raval S et al. Up-regulated p75NTR neurotrophin receptor on glial cells in MS plaques. Neurology 1999; 53: 1676–82.

639 Bonetti B, Raine CS. Multiple sclerosis: oligodendrocytes display cell death-related molecules in situ but do not undergo apoptosis. Ann Neurol 1997; 42: 74–84.

640 Wolswijk G. Oligodendrocyte regeneration in the adult rodent CNS and the failure of this process in multiple sclerosis. Prog Brain Res 1998; 117: 233–47.

641 Wolswijk G. Chronic stage multiple sclerosis lesions contain a relatively quiescent population of oligodendrocyte precursor cells. J Neurosci 1998; 18: 601–9.

642 Rice GP, Lesaux J, Vandervoort P, Macewan L, Ebers GC. Ondansetron, a 5-HT3

antagonist, improves cerebellar tremor. J Neurol Neurosurg Psychiatry 1997; 62: 282–4.

643 Optic Neuritis Study Group. The clinical profile of optic neuritis. Experience of the optic neuritis treatment trial. Arch Ophthalmol 1991; 109: 1673–8.

644 Matthews WB, Compston A, Allen IV, Martyn CN, eds. McAlpine's multiple sclerosis. Edinburgh: Churchill Livingstone, 1991: 79–105.

645 Francis DA, Compston DAS, Batchelor JR, McDonal WI. A reassessment of the risk of multiple sclerosis developing in patients with optic neuritis after extended follow up. J Neurol Neurosurg Psychiatry 1987; 50: 758–65.

646 Scholl GB, Song H.S, Wray S. Uhthoff's symptom in optic neuritis: relationship to magnetic resonance imaging and development of multiple sclerosis. Ann Neurol 1991; 30: 180–4.

647 Jacobs LD, Kaba SE, Miller CM, Priore RL, Brownscheidle CM. Correlation of clinical, magnetic resonance imaging, and cerebrospinal fluid findings in optic neuritis. Ann Neurol 1997; 41: 392–8.

648 Optic Neuritis Study Group. The 5-year risk of MS after optic neuritis. Experience of the optic neuritis treatment trial. Neurology 1997; 49: 1404–13.

649 Jin YP, de Pedro-Cuesta J, Soderstrom M, Stawiarz L, Link H. Incidence of optic neuritis in Stockholm, Sweden 1990–1995: I. Age, sex, birth and ethnic-group related patterns. J Neurol Sci 1998; 159: 107–14.

650 Ghezzi A, Martinelli V, Torri V et al. Long-term follow-up of isolated optic neuritis: the risk of developing multiple sclerosis, its outcome, and the prognostic role of paraclinical tests. J Neurol 1999; 246: 770–5.

651 Beck RW, Arrington J, Murtagh FR, Cleary PA, Kaufman DI. Brain magnetic resonance imaging in acute optic neuritis – experience of the optic neuritis study group. Arch Neurol 1993; 50: 841–6.

652 Soderstrom M, Jin YP, Hillert J, Link H. Optic neuritis, prognosis for multiple sclerosis from MRI, CSF, and HLA findings. Neurology 1998; 50: 708–14.

653 Fukaura H, Kent SC, Pietrusewicz MJ, Khoury SJ, Weiner HL, Hafler DA. Induction of circulating myelin basic protein and proteolipid protein-specific transforming growth factor-beta1-secreting Th3 T cells by oral administration of myelin in multiple sclerosis patients. J Clin Invest 1996; 98: 70–7.

654 Francis G, Evans A, Panitch H. MRI results of a phase III trial of oral myelin in relapsing-remitting multiple sclerosis. Ann Neurol 1997; 42: 467.

655 Panitch H, Francis G, Group atOmS. Clinical results of a phase III trial of oral myelin in relapsing-remitting multiple sclerosis. Ann Neurol 1997; 42: 459.

656 Evidence of interferon beta-1a dose response in relapsing-remitting MS: the OWIMS Study. The Once Weekly Interferon for MS Study Group. Neurology 1999; 53: 679–86.

657 Hohol MJ, Guttmann CR, Orav J et al. Serial neuropsychological assessment and magnetic resonance imaging analysis in multiple sclerosis. Arch Neurol 1997; 54: 1018–25.

658 Stenager E, Knudsen L, Jensen K. Acute and chronic pain syndromes in multiple sclerosis. Acta Neurol Scand 1991; 84: 197–200.

659 Vermote R, Ketelaer P, Carton H. Pain in multiple sclerosis patients. A prospective study using the Mc Gill Pain Questionnaire. Clin Neurol Neurosurg 1986; 88: 87–93.

660 Osterman PO, Westerberg CE. Paroxysmal attacks in multiple sclerosis. Brain 1975; 98: 189–202.

661 Zeldowicz L. Paroxysmal motor episodes as early manifestations of multiple sclerosis. Can Med Ass J 1961; 84: 937–41.

662 Twomey JA, Espir MLE. Paroxysmal symptoms as the first manifestations of multiple sclerosis. J Neurol Neurosurg Psychiatry 1980; 43: 296–304.

663 Matthews WB. Paroxysmal symptoms in multiple sclerosis. J Neurol Neurosurg Psych 1975; 38: 617–23.

664 Harrison N, McGill JI. Transient neurological disturbances in disseminated sclerosis: a case report. J Neurol Neurosurg Psychiatry 1969; 32: 230–2.

665 Schapiro RT, Baumhefner RW, Tourtellotte WW. Multiple sclerosis: a clinical view-

point to management. In: Multiple Sclerosis, Clinical and Pathogenetic Basis. Raine CS, McFarland HF, Tourtellotte WW, eds. London: Chapman & Hall Medical, 1997: 391–420.

666 Solaro C, Lunardi GL, Capello E et al. An open-label trial of gabapentin treatment of paroxysmal symptoms in multiple sclerosis patients. Neurology 1998; 51: 609–11.

667 Krupp LB, Coyle PK, Cross AH. Amelioration of fatigue with pemoline in patients with multiple sclerosis. Ann Neurol 1989; 26: 155–6.

668 Weinshenker BG, Penman M, Bass B, Ebers GC, Rice GP. A double-blind, random-ized, crossover trial of pemoline in fatigue associated with multiple sclerosis. Neurology 1992; 42: 1468–71.

669 Rieckmann P, Weber F, Gunther A et al. Pentoxifylline, a phosphodiesterase inhibitor, induces immune deviation in patients with multiple sclerosis. J Neuroimmunol 1996; 64: 193–200.

670 van Oosten BW, Rep MH, van Lier RA et al. A pilot study investigating the effects of orally administered pentoxifylline on selected immune variables in patients with multiple sclerosis. J Neuroimmunol 1996; 66: 49–55.

671 Myers LW, Ellison GW, Merrill JE et al. Pentoxifylline is not a promising treatment for multiple sclerosis in progression phase. Neurology 1998; 51: 1483–6.

672 Rieckmann P, Weber F, Gunther A, Poser S. The phosphodiesterase inhibitor pentox-ifylline reduces early side effects of interferon–beta 1b treatment in patients with multiple sclerosis. Neurology 1996; 47: 604.

673 Shaw PJ, Smith NM, Ince PG, Bates D. Chronic periphlebitis retinae in multiple sclerosis. A histopathological study. J Neurol Sci 1987; 77: 147–52.

674 Dau PC, Petajan JH, Johnson KP, Panitch HS, Bornstein MB. Plasmapheresis in mul-tiple sclerosis: preliminary findings. Neurology 1980; 30: 1023–8.

675 Khatri BO, McQuillen MP, Harrington GJ, Schmoll D, Hoffmann RG. Chronic pro-gressive multiple sclerosis: double-blind controlled study of plasmapheresis in patients taking immunosuppressive drugs. Neurology 1985; 35: 312–19.

676 Khatri BO, McQuillen MP, Hoffmann RG, Harrington GJ, Schmoll D. Plasma exchange in chronic progressive multiple sclerosis: a long-term study. Neurology 1991; 41: 409–14.

677 Gordon PA, Carroll DJ, Etches WS et al. A double-blind controlled pilot study of plasma exchange versus sham apheresis in chronic progressive multiple sclerosis. Can J Neurol Sci 1985; 12: 39–44.

678 Sorensen PS, Wanscher B, Szpirt W et al. Plasma exchange combined with azathio-prine in multiple sclerosis using serial gadolinium-enhanced MRI to monitor disease activity: a randomized single-masked cross-over pilot study. Neurology 1996; 46: 1620–5.

679 Vamvakas EC, Pineda AA, Weinshenker BG. Meta-analysis of clinical studies of the efficacy of plasma exchange in the treatment of chronic progressive multiple scler-osis. J Clin Apheresis 1995; 10: 163–70.

680 Weinshenker BG, O'Brien PC, Petterson TM et al. A randomised trial of plasma exchange in acute central nervous system inflammatory demyelinating disease. Ann Neurol 1999; 46: 878–86.

681 Zeek PM. Periarteritis nodosa – a critical review. Am J Clin Pathol 1952; 22: 777–90.

682 Dworkin RH, Bates D, Millar JH, Paty DW. Linoleic acid and multiple sclerosis: a reanalysis of three double-blind trials. Neurology 1984; 34: 1441–5.

683 Swank RL, Dugan BB. Effect of low saturated fat diet in early and late cases of mul-tiple sclerosis. Lancet 1990; 336: 37–9.

684 Kurtzke JF, Hyllested K. Multiple sclerosis in the Faroe Islands: II. Clinical update, transmission, and the nature of MS. Neurology 1986; 36: 307–28.

685 Kurtzke JF, Hyllested K. Multiple sclerosis in the Faroe Islands: I. Clinical and epi-demiological features. Ann Neurol 1979; 5: 6–21

686 Kurtzke JF, Hyllested K. Validity of the epidemics of multiple sclerosis in the Faroe Islands. Neuroepidemiology 1988; 7: 190–227.

687 Kurtzke J.F. Epidemiologic evidence for multiple sclerosis as an infection. Clin Microbiol Rev 1993; 6: 382–427.

688 Ingalls TH. Clustering of multiple sclerosis in Galion, Ohio, 1982–1985. Am J Forensic Med Pathol 1989; 10: 213–15.

689 Helmick CG, Wrigley JM, Zack MM et al. Multiple sclerosis in Key West, Florida. Am J Epidemiol 1989; 130: 935–49.

690 Hader WJ, Irvine DG, Schiefer HB. A cluster-focus of multiple sclerosis at Henribourg, Saskatchewan. Can J Neurol Sci 1990; 17: 391–4.

691 Barnes D, Hughes RA, Morris RW et al. Randomised trial of oral and intravenous methylprednisolone in acute relapses of multiple sclerosis. Lancet 1997; 349: 902–6.

692 Kurtzke JF. A reassessment of the distribution of multiple sclerosis. Part one. Acta Neurol Scand 1975; 51: 110–36.

693 Kurtzke J.F. A reassessment of the distribution of multiple sclerosis. Part two. Acta Neurol Scand 1975; 51: 137–57.

694 Kurtzke J.F. Geography in multiple sclerosis. J Neurol 1977; 215: 1–26.

695 Rosati G. Descriptive epidemiology of multiple sclerosis in Europe in the 1980s: a critical overview. Ann Neurol 1994; 36(Suppl 2): S164–74.

696 Page WF, Kurtzke JF, Murphy FM, Norman JE. Epidemiology of multiple sclerosis in U.S. veterans: V. Ancestry and the risk of multiple sclerosis. Ann Neurol 1993; 33: 632–9.

697 Hammond SR, McLeod JG, Millingen KS et al. The epidemiology of multiple sclerosis in three Australian cities: Perth, Newcastle and Hobart. Brain 1988; 111: 1–25.

698 Ebers GC, Sadovnick AD. The geographic distribution of multiple sclerosis: a review. Neuroepidemiology 1993; 12: 1–5.

699 Kurtzke JF, Hyllested K. Multiple sclerosis in the Faroe Islands. III. An alternative assessment of the three epidemics. Acta Neurol Scand 1987; 76: 317–39.

700 Bashir K, Whitaker JN. Clinical and laboratory features of primary progressive and secondary progressive MS. Neurology 1999; 53: 765–71.

701 Thompson AJ, Montalban X, Barkhof F et al. Diagnostic criteria for primary progressive multiple sclerosis: a position paper. Ann Neurol 2000; 47: 831–5.

702 Shirazi Y, Rus HG, Macklin WB, Shin ML. Enhanced degradation of messenger RNA encoding myelin proteins by terminal complement complexes in oligodendrocytes. J Immunol 1993; 150: 4581–90.

703 Hilliyard SA, Kutas M. Electrophisiology of cognitive processing. Annu Rev Psychol 1983; 34: 33–61.

704 Feinstein A, du Boulay G, Ron MA. Psychotic illness in multiple sclerosis, a clinical and magnetic resonance imaging study. Br J Psychiatry 1992; 161: 680–5.

705 Ritvo PG, Fischer JS, Miller DM et al. Multiple Sclerosis Quality of Life Inventory (MSQLI): a user's manual. New York: National Multiple Sclerosis Society, 1997.

706 Cohen L, Pouwer F, Pfennings LE et al. Factor structure of the Disability and Impact Profile in patients with multiple sclerosis. Qual Life Res 1999; 8: 141–50.

707 Baumhefner RW, Tourtellotte WW, Syndulko K, et al. Quantitative multiple sclerosis plaque assessment with magnetic resonance imaging. Its correlation with clinical parameters, evoked potentials, and intra-blood-brain barrier IgG synthesis. Arch Neurol 1990; 47: 19–26.

708 Poser CM. Viking voyages: the origin of multiple sclerosis? An essay in medical history. Acta Neurol Scand Suppl 1995; 161: 11–22.

709 Hobart JC, Lamping DL, Thompson AJ. Evaluating neurological outcome measures: the bare essentials. J Neurol Neurosurg Psychiatry 1996; 60: 127–30.

710 Lucchinetti CF, Bruck W, Rodriguez M, Lassmann H. Distinct patterns of multiple sclerosis pathology indicates heterogeneity on pathogenesis. Brain Pathol 1996; 6: 259–74.

711 Lassmann H, Bruck W, Lucchinetti C, Rodriguez M. Remyelination in multiple sclerosis. Mult Scler 1997; 3: 133–6.

712 Linington C, Engelhardt B, Kapocs G, Lassman H. Induction of persistently demyelinated lesions in the rat following the repeated adoptive transfer of encephalitogenic T cells and demyelinating antibody. J Neuroimmunol 1992; 40: 219–24.

713 Rodriguez M, Lennon VA. Immunoglobulins promote remyelination in the central nervous system. Ann Neurol 1990; 27: 12–17.

714 Kalkers NF, Barkhof F, Bergers E et al. The effect of neuroprotective agent riluzole on MRI parameters in primary progressive multiple sclerosis: a pilot study. Mult Scler 2002; 8: 532–3.

715 Lehmann D, Karussis D, Mizrachi-Koll R, Linde AS, Abramsky O. Inhibition of the progression of multiple sclerosis by linomide is associated with upregulation of CD4+/CD45RA+ cells and downregulation of CD4+/CD45RO+ cells. Clin Immunol Immunopathol 1997; 85: 202–9.

716 Andersen O, Lycke J, Tollesson PO et al. Linomide reduces the rate of active lesions in relapsing-remitting multiple sclerosis. Neurology 1996; 47: 895–900.

717 Karussis DM, Meiner Z, Lehmann D et al. Treatment of secondary progressive multiple sclerosis with the immunomodulator linomide: a double-blind, placebo-controlled pilot study with monthly magnetic resonance imaging evaluation. Neurology 1996; 47: 341–6.

718 Tian WZ, Navikas V, Matusevicius D et al. Linomide (roquinimex) affects the balance between pro- and anti-inflammatory cytokines in vitro in multiple sclerosis. Acta Neurol Scand 1998; 98: 94–101.

719 Tan IL, Lycklama a Nijeholt GJ, Polman CH, Ader HJ, Barkhof F. Linomide in the treatment of multiple sclerosis: MRI results from prematurely terminated phase-III trials. Mult Scler 2000; 6: 99–104.

720 Missler U, Wandinger KP, Wiesmann M, Kaps M, Wessel K. Acute exacerbation of multiple sclerosis increases plasma levels of S-100 protein. Acta Neurol Scand 1997; 96: 142–4.

721 Lassmann H, Vass K. Are current immunological concepts of multiple sclerosis reflected by the immunopathology of its lesions? Springer Semin Immunopathol 1995; 17: 77–87.

722 Huxley AF, Stamfli R. Evidence for saltatory conduction in peripheral myelinated nerve fibres. J Physiol 1949; 108: 316–39.

723 Stern BJ, Krumholz A, Johns C, Scott P, Nissim J. Sarcoidosis and its neurological manifestations. Arch Neurol 1985; 42: 909–17.

724 Miller DH, Kendall BE, Barter S et al. Magnetic resonance imaging in central nervous system sarcoidosis. Neurology 1988; 38: 378–83.

725 Nosal A, Schleissner LA, Mishkin FS, Lieberman J. Angiotensin-I-converting enzyme and gallium scan in noninvasive evaluation of sarcoidosis. Ann Intern Med 1979; 90: 328–31.

726 Pretorius ML, Loock DB, Ravenscroft A, Schoeman JF. Demyelinating disease of Schilder type in three young South African children: dramatic response to corticosteroids. J Child Neurol 1998; 13: 197–201.

727 Fitzgerald MJ, Coleman LT. Recurrent myelinoclastic diffuse sclerosis: a case report of a child with Schilder's variant of multiple sclerosis. Pediatr Radiol 2000; 30: 861–5.

728 Schilder P. Zur Kenntnis der diffusen Sklerose. Z Ges Neurol Psychiat 1912; 10: 1–60.

729 Poser CM, Goutieres F, Carpentier MA, Aicardi J. Schilder's myelinoclastic diffuse sclerosis. Pediatrics 1986; 77: 107–12.

730 Garell PC, Menezes AH, Baumbach G et al. Presentation, management and follow-up of Schilder's disease. Pediatr Neurosurg 1998; 29: 86–91.

731 Ruggieri M, Polizzi A, Pavone L, Grimaldi LM. Multiple sclerosis in children under 6 years of age. Neurology 1999; 53: 478–84.

732 Afifi AK, Bell WE, Menezes AH, Moore SA. Myelinoclastic diffuse sclerosis (Schilder's disease): report of a case and review of the literature. J Child Neurol 1994; 9: 398–403.

733 Koziol JA, Frutos A, Sipe JC, Romine JS, Beutler E. A comparison of two neurologic scoring instruments for multiple sclerosis. J Neurol 1996; 243: 209–13.

734 Confavreux C, Aimard G, Devic M. Course and prognosis of multiple sclerosis assessed by the computerized data processing of 349 patients. Brain 1980; 103: 281–300.

735 Duquette P, Murray TJ, Pleines J et al. Multiple sclerosis in childhood: clinical profile in 125 patients. J Pediatr 1987; 111: 359–63.

191

736 Robertson N, Compston A. Surveying multiple sclerosis in the United Kingdom. J Neurol Neurosurg Psychiatry 1995; 58: 2–6.

737 Minderhoud JM, Leemkius JG, Kremer J, Jaban E, Smits PML. Sexual disturbances arising from multiple sclerosis. Acta Neurol Scand 1984; 70: 299–306.

738 Dewis ME, Thornton NG. Sexual dysfunction in multiple sclerosis. J Neurol Nursing 1989; 21: 175–9.

739 Betts CD, Jones SJ, Fowler CG, Fowler CJ. Erectile dysfunction in multiple sclerosis. Associated neurological deficits, and treatment of the condition. Brain 1994; 117: 1303–10.

740 Schlesinger H. Zur Frage der akuten multiplen Sklerose und der encephalomyelitis disseminata im Kindesalter. Arb Neurol Inst (Wien) 1909; 17: 410–32.

741 Gass A, Moseley IF, Barker GJ et al. Lesion discrimination in optic neuritis using high-resolution fat-suppressed fast spin-echo MRI. Neuroradiology 1996; 38: 317–21.

742 Miller DH, Newton MR, van der Poel JC et al. Magnetic resonance imaging of the optic nerve in optic neuritis. Neurology 1988; 38: 175–9.

743 Alexander EL, Malinow K, Lejewski JE et al. Primary Sjogren's syndrome with central nervous system disease mimicking multiple sclerosis. Ann Intern Med 1986; 104: 323–30.

744 Alexander EL, Beall SS, Gordon B et al. Magnetic resonance imaging of cerebral lesions in patients with the Sjogren syndrome. Ann Intern Med 1988; 108: 815–23.

745 Hakala M, Niemela RK. Does autonomic nervous impairment have a role in pathophysiology of Sjogren's syndrome. Lancet 2000; 355: 1032–3.

746 Numer MR. Evoked potentials in multiple sclerosis. In: Raine CS, McFarland HF, Tourtellotte WW, eds. Multiple Sclerosis, Clinical and Pathogenetic Basis. London: Chapman & Hall Medical, 1997: 43–55.

747 Gronseth GS, Ashman EJ. Practice parameter: the usefulness of evoked potentials in identifying clinically silent lesions in patients with suspected multiple sclerosis (an evidence-based review): Report of the Quality Standards Subcommittee of the American Academy of Neurology. Neurology 2000; 54: 1720–5.

748 Riise T, Gronning M, Klauber MR et al. Clustering of residence of multiple sclerosis patients at age 13 to 20 years in Hordaland, Norway. Am J Epidemiol 1991; 133: 932–9.

749 Lance J.W. Symposium synopsis. In: Spasticity: disordered motor control. Feldman RG, Young RR, Koella WP, eds. Chicago: Year Book Medical Publishers, 1980: 485–94.

750 SPECTRIMS. Randomized controlled trial of interferon-beta-1a in secondary progressive MS: Clinical results. Neurology 2001; 56: 1496–504.

751 Li DK, Zhao GJ, Paty DW. Randomized controlled trial of interferon-beta-1a in secondary progressive MS: MRI results. Neurology 2001; 56: 1505–13.

752 van Noort JM, van Sechel AC, Bajramovic JJ et al. The small heat-shock protein alpha B-crystallin as candidate autoantigen in multiple sclerosis. Nature 1995; 375: 798–801.

753 Selmaj K, Brosnan CF, Raine CS. Expression of heat shock protein–65 by oligodendrocytes in vivo and in vitro: implications for multiple sclerosis. Neurology 1992; 42: 795–800.

754 Aquino DA, Capello E, Weisstein J et al. Multiple sclerosis: altered expression of 70- and 27-kDa heat shock proteins in lesions and myelin. J Neuropathol Exp Neurol 1997; 56: 664–72.

755 Yu JS, Hayashi T, Seboun E et al. Fos RNA accumulation in multiple sclerosis white matter tissue. J Neurol Sci 1991; 103: 209–15.

756 Reynolds EH, Bottiglieri T, Laundy M, Crellin RF, Kirker SG. Vitamin B12 metabolism in multiple sclerosis. Arch Neurol 1992; 49: 649–52.

757 Tsubaki T, Honma Y, Hoshi M. Neurological syndrome associated with clioquinol. Lancet 1971; 1: 696–7.

758 Cummings JL, Benson DF. Subcortical dementia: review of an emerging concept. Arch Neurol 1984; 41: 874–9.

759 Rao SM. Neuropsychology of multiple sclerosis: a critical review. J Clin Exp Neuropsychol 1986; 8: 503–42.

760 Cummings JL. Introduction. In: Subcortical Dementia. Cummings JL, ed. New York: Oxford University Press, 1990: 3–16.

761 Sadovnick AD, Dircks A, Ebers GC. Genetic counselling in multiple sclerosis: risks to sibs and children of affected individuals. Clin Genet 1999; 56: 118–22.

762 Stenager EN, Stenager E, Koch-Henriksen N et al. Suicide and multiple sclerosis. J Neurol Neurosurg Psychiatry 1992; 55: 542–5.

763 Peppercorn MA. Sulfasalazine. Pharmacology, clinical use, toxicity, and related new drug development. Ann Intern Med 1984; 101: 377–86.

764 Noseworthy JH, O'Brien P, Erickson BJ et al. The Mayo Clinic-Canadian Cooperative trial of sulfasalazine in active multiple sclerosis. Neurology 1998; 51: 1342–52.

765 Young H. Syphilis. Serology. Dermatol Clin 1998; 16: 691–8.

766 Winfield JB, Shaw M, Silverman LM et al. Intrathecal IgG synthesis and blood-brain barrier impairment in patients with systemic lupus erythematosus and central nervous system dysfunction. Am J Med 1983; 74: 837–44.

767 Ormerod IE, Miller DH, McDonald WI et al. The role of NMR imaging in the assessment of multiple sclerosis and isolated neurological lesions. A quantitative study. Brain 1987; 110: 1579–616.

768 Barned S, Goodman AD, Mattson DH. Frequency of anti-nuclear antibodies in multiple sclerosis. Neurology 1995; 45: 384–5.

769 Isshi K, Hirohata S. Differential roles of the anti-ribosomal P antibody and antineuronal antibody in the pathogenesis of central nervous system involvement in systemic lupus erythematosus. Arthritis Rheum 1998; 41: 1819–27.

770 Bell RB, Ramachandran S. The relationship of TAP1 and TAP2 dimorphisms to multiple sclerosis susceptibility. J Neuroimmunol 1995; 59: 201–4.

771 Bennetts BH, Teutsch SM, Heard RN, Dunckley H, Stewart GJ. TAP2 polymorphisms in Australian multiple sclerosis patients. J Neuroimmunol 1995; 59: 113–21.

772 Wekerle H. Immunology of multiple sclerosis. In: Compston A, Ebers G, Lassmann H, McDonald I, Matthews B, Wekerle H, eds. Multiple Sclerosis. Edinburgh: Churchill Livingstone, 1998: 379–407.

773 Hashimoto LL, Mak TW, Ebers GC. T cell receptor alpha chain polymorphisms in multiple sclerosis. J Neuroimmunol 1992; 40: 41–8.

774 Lynch SG, Rose JW, Petajan JH, Leppert M. Discordance of the T-cell receptor alpha-chain gene in familial multiple sclerosis. Neurology 1992; 42: 839–44.

775 Eoli M, Wood NW, Kellar-Wood HF et al. No linkage between multiple sclerosis and the T cell receptor alpha chain locus. J Neurol Sci 1994; 124: 32–7.

776 Hillert J, Leng C, Olerup O. No association with germline T cell receptor beta-chain gene alleles or haplotypes in Swedish patients with multiple sclerosis. J Neuroimmunol 1991; 32: 141–7.

777 Vandevyver C, Buyse I, Philippaerts L et al. HLA and T-cell receptor polymorphisms in Belgian multiple sclerosis patients: no evidence for disease association with the T-cell receptor. J Neuroimmunol 1994; 52: 25–32.

778 Leonard JP, Waldburger KE, Goldman SJ. Prevention of experimental autoimmune encephalomyelitis by antibodies against interleukin 12. J Exp Med 1995; 181: 381–6.

779 Voskuhl RR, Martin R, Bergman C et al. T helper 1 (Th1) functional phenotype of human myelin basic protein-specific T lymphocytes. Autoimmunity 1993; 15: 137–43.

780 Druet P, Sheela R, Pelletier L. Th1 and Th2 cells in autoimmunity. Clin Exp Immunol 1995; 101(Suppl 1): 9–12.

781 Laman JD, Thompson EJ, Kappos L. Balancing the Th1/Th2 concept in multiple sclerosis. Immunol Today 1998; 19: 489–90.

782 Sornasse T, Larenas PV, Davis KA, de Vries JE, Yssel H. Differentiation and stability of T helper 1 and 2 cells derived from naive human neonatal CD4+ T cells, analyzed at the single-cell level. J Exp Med 1996; 184: 473–83.

783 Constantinescu CS, Hilliard B, Ventura E et al. Modulation of susceptibility and resistance to an autoimmune model of multiple sclerosis in prototypically susceptible and

resistant strains by neutralization of interleukin-12 and interleukin-4, respectively. Clin Immunol 2001; 98: 23–30.

784 Chen Y, Kuchroo VK, Inobe J, Hafler DA, Weiner HL. Regulatory T cell clones induced by oral tolerance: suppression of autoimmune encephalomyelitis. Science 1994; 265: 1237–40.

785 Larsson HB, Frederiksen J, Kjaer L, Henriksen O, Olesen J. In vivo determination of T1 and T2 in the brain of patients with severe but stable multiple sclerosis. Magn Reson Med 1988; 7: 43–55.

786 Ormerod IE, Johnson G, MacManus D, du Boulay EP, McDonald WI. Relaxation times of apparently normal cerebral white matter in multiple sclerosis. Acta Radiol Suppl 1986; 369: 382–4.

787 Barnes D, Munro PM, Youl BD, Prineas JW, McDonald WI. The longstanding MS lesion. A quantitative MRI and electron microscopic study. Brain 1991; 114: 1271–80.

788 Kidd D, Barker GJ, Tofts PS et al. The transverse magnetisation decay characteristics of longstanding lesions and normal-appearing white matter in multiple sclerosis. J Neurol 1997; 244: 125–30.

789 Armspach JP, Gounot D, Rumbach L, Chambron J. In vivo determination of multi-exponential T2 relaxation in the brain of patients with multiple sclerosis. Magn Reson Imaging 1991; 9: 107–13.

790 MacKay A, Whittall K, Adler J et al. In vivo visualization of myelin water in brain by magnetic resonance. Magn Reson Med 1994; 31: 673–7.

791 Rao SM. Cognitive Function Study Group, National Multiple Sclerosis Society. Manual for the Brief Repeatable Battery of Neuropsychological Tests in Multiple Sclerosis. New York: National Multiple Sclerosis Society, 1990.

792 Thompson AJ, Hobart JC. Multiple sclerosis: assessment of disability and disability scales. J Neurol 1998; 245: 189–96.

793 Smith C, Birnbaum G, Carter JL, Greenstein J, Lublin FD. Tizanidine treatment of spasticity caused by multiple sclerosis: results of a double-blind, placebo-controlled trial. US Tizanidine Study Group. Neurology 1994; 44(11)(Suppl 9): S34–42; discussion S42–43.

794 UKTTG. A double-blind, placebo-controlled trial of tizanidine in the treatment of spasticity caused by multiple sclerosis. United Kingdom Tizanidine Trial Group. Neurology 1994; 44: S70–8.

795 Nance PW, Sheremata WA, Lynch SG et al. Relationship of the antispasticity effect of tizanidine to plasma concentration in patients with multiple sclerosis. Arch Neurol 1997; 54: 731–6.

796 Stien R, Nordal HJ, Oftedal SI, Slettebo M. The treatment of spasticity in multiple sclerosis: a double-blind clinical trial of a new anti-spastic drug tizanidine compared with baclofen. Acta Neurol Scand 1987; 75: 190–4.

797 Shibasaki H, Kuroiwa Y. Painful tonic seizures in multiple sclerosis. Arch Neurol 1974; 30: 47–51.

798 Filipi M, Horsfield MA, Morrisey SP et al. Quantitative brain MRI lesion load predicts the course of clinically isolated syndromes suggestive of multiple sclerosis. Neurology 1994; 44: 635–41.

799 Wahl SM. Transforming growth factor beta: the good, the bad, and the ugly. J Exp Med 1994; 180: 1587–90

800 Carrieri PB, Provitera V, De Rosa T et al. Profile of cerebrospinal fluid and serum cytokines in patients with relapsing-remitting multiple sclerosis: a correlation with clinical activity. Immunopharmacol Immunotoxicol 1998; 20: 373–82.

801 Bertolotto A, Capobianco M, Malucchi S et al. Transforming growth factor beta1 (TGFbeta1) mRNA level correlates with magnetic resonance imaging disease activity in multiple sclerosis patients. Neurosci Lett 1999; 263: 21–4.

802 Nicoletti F, Di Marco R, Patti F et al. Blood levels of transforming growth factor-beta 1 (TGF-beta1) are elevated in both relapsing remitting and chronic progressive multiple sclerosis (MS) patients and are further augmented by treatment with interferon-beta 1b (IFN-beta1b). Clin Exp Immunol 1998; 113: 96–9.

803 Ossege LM, Sindern E, Patzold T, Malin JP. Immunomodulatory effects of interferon-beta-1b in vivo: induction of the expression of transforming growth factor-beta1 and its receptor type II. J Neuroimmunol 1998; 91: 73–81.

804 Calabresi PA, Fields NS, Maloni HW et al. Phase 1 trial of transforming growth factor beta 2 in chronic progressive MS. Neurology 1998; 51: 289–92.

805 Scott TF, Bhagavatula K, Snyder PJ, Chieffe C. Transverse myelitis. Comparison with spinal cord presentations of multiple sclerosis. Neurology 1998; 50: 429–33.

806 Weinshenker BG, Bass B, Karlik S, Ebers GC, Rice GP. An open trial of OKT3 in patients with multiple sclerosis. Neurology 1991; 41: 1047–52.

807 Albert PS, McFarland HF, Smith ME, Frank JA. Time series for modelling counts from a relapsing-remitting disease: application to modelling disease activity in multiple sclerosis. Stat Med 1994; 13: 453–66.

808 Confavreux C, Vukusic S, Grimaud J, Moreau T. Clinical progression and decision making process in multiple sclerosis. Mult Scler 1999; 5: 212–15.

809 Jensen TS, Rasmussen P, Reske-Nielsen E. Association of trigeminal neuralgia with multiple sclerosis: clinical and pathological features. Acta Neurol Scand 1982; 38: 1830–4.

810 Gaur A, Fathman CG. Immunotherapeutic strategies directed at the trimolecular complex. Adv Immunol 1994; 56: 219–65.

811 Kuroda Y, Shimamoto Y. Human tumor necrosis factor-alpha augments experimental allergic encephalomyelitis in rats. J Neuroimmunol 1991; 34: 159–64.

812 Hofman FM, Hinton DR, Johnson K, Merrill JE. Tumor necrosis factor identified in multiple sclerosis brain. J Exp Med 1989; 170: 607–12.

813 Maimone D, Gregory S, Arnason BG, Reder AT. Cytokine levels in the cerebrospinal fluid and serum of patients with multiple sclerosis. J Neuroimmunol 1991; 32: 67–74.

814 Sharief MK, Hentges R. Association between tumor necrosis factor-alpha and disease progression in patients with multiple sclerosis. N Engl J Med 1991; 325: 467–72.

815 van Oosten BW, Barkhof F, Scholten PE et al. Increased production of tumor necrosis factor alpha, and not of interferon gamma, preceding disease activity in patients with multiple sclerosis. Arch Neurol 1998; 55: 793–8.

816 Selmaj K, Raine CS, Cross AH. Anti-tumour necrosis factor therapy abrogates autoimmune demyelination. Ann Neurol 1991; 30: 694–700.

817 Frei K, Eugster HP, Bopst M et al. Tumor necrosis factor alpha and lymphotoxin alpha are not required for induction of acute experimental autoimmune encephalomyelitis. J Exp Med 1997; 185: 2177–82.

818 Gayo A, Mozo L, Suarez A et al. Interferon beta-1b treatment modulates TNFalpha and IFNgamma spontaneous gene expression in MS. Neurology 1999; 52: 1764–70.

819 Roth MP, Nogueira L, Coppin H et al. Tumor necrosis factor polymorphism in multiple sclerosis: no additional association independent of HLA. J Neuroimmunol 1994; 51: 93–9.

820 He B, Navikas V, Lundahl J, Soderstrom M, Hillert J. Tumor necrosis factor alpha-308 alleles in multiple sclerosis and optic neuritis. J Neuroimmunol 1995; 63: 143–7.

821 Wingerchuk D, Liu Q, Sobell J et al. A population-based case-control study of the tumour necrosis factor alpha-308 polymorphism in multiple sclerosis. Neurology 1997; 49: 626–8.

822 Yousry TA, Filippi M, Becker C, Horsfield MA, Voltz R. Comparison of MR pulse sequences in the detection of multiple sclerosis lesions. AJNR 1997; 18: 959–63.

823 Kurtzke JF, Hyllested K, Helrberg A, Olsen A. Multiple sclerosis in the Faroe Islands. The occurrence of the fourth epidemic as validation of transmission. Acta Neurol Scand 1993; 88: 161–73.

824 Persson HE, Sachs C. Visual evoked potentials elicited by pattern reversal during provoked visual impairment in multiple sclerosis. Brain 1981; 104: 369–82.

825 Hays RD, Steward AL. Construct validity of MOS health measures. In: Stewart AL, Ware JEJ, eds. The medical outcomes study approach. Durham, NC: Duke University Press, 1993: 325–45.

826 Stewart AL, Hays RD, Ware JEJ. Methods of validating MOS health measures. In:

195

Stewart AL, Ware JEJ, eds. Measuring functioning and well-being. Durham, NC: Duke University Press, 1993: 309–25.

827 Elices MJ, Osborn L, Takada Y et al. VCAM-1 on activated endothelium interacts with the leukocyte integrin VLA-4 at a site distinct from the VLA-4/fibronectin binding site. Cell 1990; 60: 577–84.

828 Wakefield AJ, More LJ, Difford J, McLaughlin JE. Immunohistochemical study of vascular injury in acute multiple sclerosis. J Clin Pathol 1994; 47: 129–33.

829 Martinelli V, Comi G, Filippi M et al. Paraclinical tests in acute-onset optic neuritis: basal data and results of a short follow-up. Acta Neurol Scand 1991; 84: 231–6.

830 Nikoskelainen E, Reikkenen P. Optic neuritis: a sign of multiple sclerosis or other diseases of the central nervous system. Acta Neurol Scand 1974; 50: 690–718.

831 Fang JP, Donahue SP, Lin RH. Global visual field involvement in acute unilateral optic neuritis. Am J Ophthalmol 1999; 128: 554–65.

832 Fang JP, Lin RH, Donahue SP. Recovery of visual field function in the Optic Neuritis Treatment Trial. Am J Ophthalmol 1999; 128: 566–72.

833 Bjartmar C, Trapp BD. Axonal and neuronal degeneration in multiple sclerosis: mechanisms and functional consequences. Curr Opin Neurol 2001; 14: 271–8.

834 McPherson D, Starr A. auditory evoked potentials in the clinic. In: Halliday AM, ed. Evoked Potentials in Clinical Testing. Edinburgh: Churchill Livingstone, 1993: 359–81.

835 Baddeley A. Working memory. Science 1992; 255: 556–9.

836 Grigsby J, Ayarbe SD, Kravcisin N, Busenbark D. Working memory impairment among persons with chronic progressive multiple sclerosis. J Neurol 1994; 241: 125–31.

837 Rao SM. Neuropsychology of multiple sclerosis. Curr Opin Neurol 1995; 8: 216–20.

838 Weinshenker BG, Issa M, Baskerville J. Long-term and short-term outcome of multiple sclerosis: a 3-year follow-up study. Arch Neurol 1996; 53: 353–8.

839 Panitch H, Goodin DS, Francis G et al. Randomized, comparative study of interferon β-1a treatment regimens in MS: The EVIDENCE Trial. Neurology 2002; 59: 1496–506.

840 Zhang JZ, Rivera VM, Tejada-Simon MV et al. T cell vaccination in multiple sclerosis: results of a preliminary study. J Neurology 2002; 249: 212–18.

841 Brownall B, Hughes. The distribution of plaques in the cerebrum in multiple sclerosis. J Neurol Neurosurg Psychiatry 1962; 25: 315–20.

842 Paty D. Interferon beta-1b. In: Hawkins CP, Wolinsky JS, eds. Principles of Treatments in Multiple Sclerosis. Oxford: Butterworth Heinemann, 2000: 24–37.

843 Purves D, Augustine GJ, Fitzpatrick D et al., eds. Neuroscience. Sunderland, MA, USA: Sinauer Associates Inc. Publishers, 1997.

844 Poser CM, ed. An Atlas of Multiple Sclerosis. London: Parthenon Publishing, 1998.

Appendices

1. EXPANDED DISABILITY STATUS SCALE (EDSS)

2. SCRIPPS NEUROLOGICAL RATING SCALE (SNRS)

3. AMBULATION INDEX (AI)

4. MULTIPLE SCLEROSIS FUNCTIONAL COMPOSITE MEASURE (MSFC)—
   GENERAL INSTRUCTIONS

5. THE GUY'S NEUROLOGICAL DISABILITY SCALE (GNDS)

6. THE MOS 36-ITEM SHORT FORM HEALTH SURVEY (SF-36)

7. FARMER QUALITY OF LIFE SCALE

8. MULTIPLE SCLEROSIS QUALITY OF LIFE (MSQOL)-54 INSTRUMENT

9. THE FAMS QUALITY OF LIFE INSTRUMENT

Appendix 1

EXPANDED DISABILITY STATUS SCALE (EDSS)

A. FUNCTIONAL SYSTEMS

Pyramidal Functions

0. Normal.
1. Abnormal signs without disability.
2. Minimal disability.
3. Mild or moderate paraparesis or hemiparesis; severe monoparesis.
4. Marked paraparesis or hemiparesis; moderate quadriparesis; or monoplegia.
5. Paraplegia, hemiplegia, or marked quadriparesis.
6. Quadriplegia.
V. Unknown.

Cerebellar Functions

0. Normal.
1. Abnormal signs without disability.
2. Mild ataxia.
3. Moderate truncal or limb ataxia.
4. Severe ataxia, all limbs.
5. Unable to perform coordinated movements due to ataxia.
V. Unknown.
X. Is used throughout after each number when weakness (grade 3 or more on pyramidal) interferes with testing.

Brain Stem Functions

0. Normal.
1. Signs only.
2. Moderate nystagmus or other mild disability.
3. Severe nystagmus, marked extraocular weakness, or moderate disability of other cranial nerves.
4. Marked dysarthria or other marked disability.
5. Inability to swallow or speak.
V. Unknown.

Reproduced by permission from Kurtzke JF. Rating neurological impairment in multiple sclerosis: an expanded disability status scale (EDSS). *Neurology* 1983; 33: 1444–52.

Sensory Functions (revised 1982)

0. Normal.
1. Vibration or figure-writing decrease only, in one or two limbs.
2. Mild decrease in touch or pain or position sense, and/or moderate decrease in vibration in one or two limbs; or vibratory (c/s figure writing) decrease alone in three or four limbs.
3. Moderate decrease in touch or pain or position sense, and/or essentially lost vibration in one or two limbs; or mild decrease in touch or pain and/or moderate decrease in all proprioceptive tests in three or four limbs.
4. Marked decrease in touch or pain or loss of proprioception, alone or combined, in one or two limbs; or moderate decrease in touch or pain and/or severe proprioceptive decrease in more than two limbs.
5. Loss (essentially) of sensation in one or two limbs; or moderate decrease in touch or pain and/or loss of proprioception for most of the body below the head.
6. Sensation essentially lost below the head.
V. Unknown.

Bowel and Bladder Functions (revised 1982)

0. Normal.
1. Mild urinary hesitancy, urgency, or retention.
2. Moderate hesitancy, urgency, retention of bowel or bladder, or rare urinary incontinence.
3. Frequent urinary incontinence.
4. In need of almost constant catheterization.
5. Loss of bladder function.
6. Loss of bowel and bladder function.
V. Unknown.

Visual (or Optic) Functions

0. Normal.
1. Scotoma with visual acuity (corrected) better than 20/30.
2. Worse eye with scotoma with maximal visual acuity (corrected) of 20/30 to 20/59.
3. Worse eye with large scotoma, or moderate decrease in fields, but with maximal visual acuity (corrected) of 20/60 to 20/99.
4. Worse eye with marked decrease of fields and maximal visual acuity (corrected) of 20/100 to 20/200; grade 3 plus maximal acuity of better eye of 20/60 or less.

5. Worse eye with maximal visual acuity (corrected) less than 20/200; grade 4 plus maximal acuity of better eye of 20/60 or less.
6. Grade 5 plus maximal acuity of better eye of 20/60 or less.
V. Unknown.
X. Is added to grades 0 to 6 for presence of temporal pallor.

Cerebral (or Mental) Functions
0. Normal.
1. Mood alteration only (Does not affect DSS score).
2. Mild decrease in mentation.
3. Moderate decrease in mentation.
4. Marked decrease in mentation (chronic brain syndrome—moderate).
5. Dementia or chronic brain syndrome—severe or incompetent.
V. Unknown.

Other Functions
0. None.
1. Any other neurologic findings attributed to MS (specify).
V. Unknown.

B. EXPANDED DISABILITY STATUS SCALE (EDSS)

0 = Normal neurologic exam (all grade 0 in Functional Systems [FS]; Cerebral grade 1 acceptable).
1.0 = No disability, minimal signs in one FS (ie, grade 1 excluding Cerebral grade 1).
1.5 = No disability minimal signs in more than one FS (more than one grade 1 excluding Cerebral grade 1).
2.0 = Minimal disability in one FS (one FS grade 2, others 0 or 1).
2.5 = Minimal disability in two FS (two FS grade 2, others 0 or 1).
3.0 = Moderate disability in one FS (one FS grade 3, others 0 or 1), or mild disability in three or four FS (three/four FS grade 2, others 0 to 1) though fully ambulatory.
3.5 = Fully ambulatory but with moderate disability in one FS (one grade 3) and one or two FS grade 2; or two FS grade 3; or five FS grade 2 (others 0 to 1).
4.0 = Fully ambulatory without aid, self-sufficient, up and about some 12 hours a day despite relatively severe disability consisting of one FS grade 4 (others 0 or 1), or combinations of lesser grades exceeding

limits of previous steps. Able to walk without aid or rest some 500 meters.

4.5 = fully ambulatory without aid, up and about much of the day, able to work a full day, may otherwise have some limitation of full activity or require minimal assistance; characterized by relatively severe disability, usually consisting of one FS grade 4 (others 0 to 1) or combinations of lesser grades exceeding limits of previous steps. Able to walk without aid or rest for some 300 meters.

5.0 = Ambulatory without aid or rest for about 200 meters; disability severe enough to impair full daily activities (eg, to work full day without special provisions). (Usual FS equivalents are one grade 5 alone, others 0 to 1; or combinations of lesser grades usually exceeding specifications for step 4.0.)

5.5 = Ambulatory without aid or rest for about 100 meters; disability severe enough to preclude full daily activities. (Usual FS equivalents are one grade 5 alone, others 0 or 1; or combinations of lesser grades usually exceeding those for step 4.0.)

6.0 = Intermittent or unilateral constant assistance (cane, crutch, or brace) required to walk about 100 meters with or without resting. (Usual FS equivalents are combinations with more than two FS grade 3+.)

6.5 = Constant bilateral assistance (canes, crutches, or braces) required to walk about 20 meters without resting. (Usual FS equivalents are combinations with more than two FS grade 3+.)

7.0 = Unable to walk beyond about 5 meters even with aid, essentially restricted to wheelchair; wheels self in standard wheelchair and transfers alone; up and about in w/c some 12 hours a day. (Usual FS equivalents are combinations with more than one FS grade 4+; very rarely, pyramidal grade 5 alone.)

7.5 = Unable to take more than a few steps; restricted to wheelchair; may need aid in transfer; wheels self but cannot carry on in standard wheelchair a full day; may require motorized wheelchair. (Usual FS equivalents are combinations with more than one FS grade 4+.)

8.0 = Essentially restricted to bed or chair or perambulated in wheelchair, but may be out of bed itself much of the day; retains many self-care functions; generally has effective use of arms. (Usual FS equivalents are combinations, generally grade 4+ in several systems.)

8.5 = Essentially restricted to bed much of the day; has some effective use of arm(s); retains some self-care functions. (Usual FS equivalents are combinations, generally 4+ in several systems.)

9.0 = Helpless bed patient; can communicate and eat. (Usual FS equivalents are combinations, mostly grade 4+.)

9.5 = Totally helpless bed patient; unable to communicate effectively or eat/swallow. (Usual FS equivalents are combinations, almost all grade 4+.)

10 = Death due to MS.

Appendix 2

SCRIPPS NEUROLOGIC RATING SCALE (SNRS)

A neurologic rating scale (NRS) has been developed for clinical assessment of MS patients. The scale has been tested on 250 MS patients. Assignment of the NRS score is based on assessment of each component of the neurologic examination and accurately reflects overall neurologic function. Clinical exacerbations are evident as significant deviations from baseline scores. There was close interexaminer correlation, with the range of variability no greater than 2.6%. The NRS is a simple, reliable, and sensitive scale that can be used with other objective measurements of neurologic function, such as neurophysiologic studies, in the clinical assessment of MS patients.

Neurologic rating scale (NRS). The assignment of points in the NRS directly reflects the examiner's clinical assessment of each component in the neurologic examination (Table 1). An intact system receives the full 'normal' point value, with a progressive loss in points for mild (−1; 1+), moderate (−2; 2+), or severe (−3, −4; 3+, 4+) involvement. Severe (−3; 3+) and maximal (−4; 4+) deficits are scored as severe on the NRS. A category for important subjective symptoms such as bladder, bowel, or sexual dysfunction was incorporated, because there is no simple way to measure central autonomic function. The total point distributions for the several systems are specifically weighted for common fluctuating neurologic abnormalities of MS, such as visual, motor, sensory, and cerebellar signs. Tendon reflexes and Babinski responses, more often present than other signs, are less emphasized. Disorders of cognition, affect, and mood are also included. The final score is obtained by noting the assigned points in each of the columns and adding the subtotals. A neurologically normal individual would have a score of 100 points.

Reproduced by permission from Sipe JC *et al*. A Neurologic Rating Scale (NRS) for use in multiple sclerosis. *Neurology (Cleveland)* 1984; 34: 1368–72.

Table 1 Scripps Neurological Rating Scale (SNRS) worksheet*

System Examined	Maximum Points	Normal	Degree of Impairment		
			Mild	Mod.	Severe
Mentation and Mood	10	10	7	4	0
Cranial Nerves: Visual Acuity	21	5	3	1	0
Fields, Discs, Pupils		6	4	2	0
Eye Movements		5	3	1	0
Nystagmus		5	3	1	0
Lower Cranial Nerves	5	5	3	1	0
Motor: RU	20	5	3	1	0
LU	5	3	1	0	
RL	5	3	1	0	
LL	5	3	1	0	
DTRS: UE	8	4	3	1	0
LE	4	3	1	0	
Babinski: R; L (2 ea)	4	4	—	—	0
Sensory: RU	12	3	2	1	0
LU	3	2	1	0	
RL	3	2	1	0	
LL	3	2	1	0	
Cerebellar: UE	10	5	3	1	0
LE		5	3	1	0
Gait; Trunk and Balance	10	10	7	4	0
Special Category:					
Bladder/Bowel/Sexual Dysfunction	0	0	−3	−7	−10
Totals	100				
Neurological Rating Scale Score	☐				

*Points assigned for each component of the neurologic examination are subtotaled, and points for autonomic dysfunction are subtracted, leaving the final (NRS) score.

Appendix 3

AMBULATION INDEX

0 Asymptomatic; fully active
1 Walks normally but reports fatigue that interferes with athletic or other demanding activities
2 Abnormal gait or episodic imbalance; gait disorder is noticed by family and friends; able to walk 25 feet (8 meters) in 10 seconds or less
3 Walks independently; able to walk 25 feet in 20 seconds or less
4 Requires unilateral support (cane or single crutch) to walk; walks 25 feet in 20 seconds or less
5 Requires bilateral support (canes, crutches, or walker) and walks 25 feet in 20 seconds or less; *or* requires unilateral support but needs more than 20 seconds to walk 25 feet
6 Requires bilateral support and more than 20 seconds to walk 25 feet; may use wheelchair* on occasion
7 Walking limited to several steps with bilateral support; unable to walk 25 feet; may use wheelchair* for most activities
8 Restricted to wheelchair; able to transfer self independently
9 Restricted to wheelchair; unable to transfer self independently

*The use of a wheelchair may be determined by life style and motivation. It is expected that patients in Grade 7 will use a wheelchair more frequently than those in Grades 5 or 6. Assignment of a grade in the range of 5 to 7, however, is determined by the patient's ability to walk a given distance, and not by the extent to which the patient uses a wheelchair.

Reproduced by permission from Hauser SL *et al*. Intensive immunosuppression in progressive multiple sclerosis. *N Engl J Med* 1983; 308: 173–80. Copyright © 1983 Massachusetts Medical Society. All rights reserved.

Appendix 4

MULTIPLE SCLEROSIS FUNCTIONAL COMPOSITE MEASURE (MSFC)—GENERAL INSTRUCTIONS

Many of those who will be administering the MSFC may not have had extensive experience with MS patients or with standardized testing procedures. The following instructions are provided to ensure that the MSFC is administered in a standardized manner, regardless of the examining technician's prior experience.

Note: A training videotape is available through the National Multiple Sclerosis Society. This videotape illustrates the proper conduct of each element of the MSFC. This videotape may be requested through the NMSS office in New York.

STANDARDIZING MSFC ADMINISTRATION

The MSFC should be administered as close to the beginning of a study visit as possible, but definitely before the patient does a distance walk. MSFC components should be administered in the following order:

1. Trial 1, Timed 25-Foot Walk
2. Trial 2, Timed 25-Foot Walk
3. Trial 1, Dominant Hand, 9-HPT
4. Trial 2, Dominant Hand, 9-HPT
5. Trial 1, Non-Dominant Hand, 9-HPT
6. Trial 2, Non-Dominant Hand, 9-HPT
7. PASAT-3"

Note: Some cognitive neuropsychologists also recommend completing the PASAT-2", which is administered at a faster rate, to provide additional information about information processing speed. This can be added as an option after the PASAT 3". Instructions for the PASAT 2" are included in this manual, although only the PASAT-3" is currently considered essential for inclusion in the MSFC.

An individual component of the MSFC should be discontinued only if the

Reproduced with permission from Fisher JS *et al. Administration and Scoring Manual for the Multiple Sclerosis Functional Composite Measure (MSFC).* New York: Demos Medical Publishing, 1999.

patient meets the discontinue criteria for that component. Other components should still be administered.

Instructions for each component measure should be given exactly as they appear in the manual. Translations of the instructions to be read to patients are available in some languages (French, German, Dutch, Greek, and Hebrew). As patients gain more experience with the tasks, many may want to skip the instructions or the PASAT practice trials. To ensure standardized administration, full instructions should be given for each task, and at least one practice trial should always be given for each section of the PASAT.

TESTING ENVIRONMENT

Every effort should be made to use the same testing room and the same designated area for the Timed 25-Foot Walk at every visit. It is essential that the potential for external distractions be kept to a minimum. All necessary materials (see p. 5) should be assembled prior to the patient's arrival. If the space designated for the Timed 25-Foot Walk is a public hallway, complete privacy may be impossible; however, every attempt should be made to keep the patient's path clear of obstacles (human or inanimate). No one other than the examiner and the patient should be in the testing room during 9-HPT and PASAT. Unplug the phones (or turn off their ringers), and turn off beepers (or switch to nonaudible notification). Establish some way to indicate to others that testing is in progress and you are not to be disturbed (e.g., a sign on the door stating 'TESTING IN PROGRESS—DO NOT DISTURB').

ESTABLISHING RAPPORT

The examining technician should be thoroughly familiar with all of the measures prior to their administration so that s/he can focus only on establishing rapport, observing the patient's behavior, and recording the patient's times and responses. The MSFC can be challenging for patients, so it is important to establish good rapport early on. Introduce yourself to the patient the first time you meet him or her and ask the patient how he or she prefers to be addressed. You may want to say something like, 'Hello, my name is Jane Doe, I'm a nurse here at the center and the examining technician for the study. Please call me Jane. How do you prefer to be addressed?' Query to find out if s/he prefers Mr., Mrs., Dr., first name, or a nickname. Make eye contact with the patient and speak in a friendly, yet professional, manner.

Offer to answer any questions the patient may have about the measures. Patients may ask things such as, 'What will I be doing today?' or 'How long will this take?' You may tell the patient things such as, 'I'll be testing your upper and lower extremity function as well as cognitive function,' or, 'You'll be doing three tasks today, which will take about 20 minutes to complete.'

RECORDING RESPONSES

Use a clipboard as your writing surface and hold it in such a way that the patient cannot see what you are writing. Please write legibly. Any deviation from the standard instructions due to examiner error or external interferences should be noted in the appropriate section of each Record Form. In general, any circumstances that may have affected the patient's performance should be recorded.

PROVIDING FEEDBACK TO THE PATIENT ABOUT HIS/HER PERFORMANCE

Do not provide the patient with test answers and do not indicate whether answers are correct or incorrect (either verbally or nonverbally, except on practice items. Do not give the patient direct feedback about his/her performances on any of the measures, i.e., the times on the Timed 25-Foot Walk or 9-HPT or the patient's total correct on PASAT. If the patient asks, 'How did I do?,' or something to that effect, give general encouragement and/or feedback such as, 'You gave great effort today,' or, 'I thought things ran very smoothly today.' If the patient appears distressed upon the completion of a task, it may be helpful to say something similar to, 'I can see that this test was very difficult for you. It can be a very challenging task and I appreciate how you gave your full effort.' It is important that you make all reasonable attempts to maintain the physical and emotional comfort of the patients as they complete the measures. At the completion of the visit be sure to thank the patient for his/her participation.

MATERIALS REQUIRED FOR THE MSFC

Clipboard, pens, stopwatch, cassette tape or CD player, PASAT stimulus tape, 9-HPT apparatus, Dycem (to stabilize the 9-HPT apparatus), clearly marked 25-foot line, Case Record Forms.

The 9-HPT apparatus is available through several vendors. For example, the Rolyan 9-Hole Peg Test is a one-piece molded plastic model that is distributed by Smith & Nephew, Inc. (Rehabilitation Division); One Quality Drive; PO Box 1005; Gemantown, WI 53022-8205; Phone: (800) 558-8633; FAX; (800) 545-7758. **WARNING:** Although the 9-HPT apparatus itself is well-constructed, the stopwatches provided with the 9-HPT by Smith & Nephew have been very unreliable in our experience. Consequently, we recommend obtaining a more reliable stopwatch through a sports store, psychological test publisher, or other vendor.

Dycem is recommended to anchor the 9-HPT apparatus and can be ordered through several suppliers of occupational therapy materials. For example, a 10" × 14" Dycem activity pad suitable for this purpose is available through Sammons Preston, Inc.; 4 Sammons Court; Bolingbrook, IL60440; Phone: (800) 323-5547; FAX: (800) 547-4333.

PASAT audiocassette tapes or CDs are available through: Stephen Rao, Ph. D.; Section of Neuropsychology; MCW Clinic at Froedtert; 9200 W. Wisconsin Avenue; Milwaukee, WI 53226; Phone: (414) 456-4665; e-mail: srao@mcw.edu. **WARNING:** Audiotapes stretch after 75 to 100 administrations, so timing of stimulus presentation should be checked and tapes replaced periodically. All other materials are readily available.

INSTRUCTIONS FOR THE TIMED 25-FOOT WALK

DESCRIPTION
The Timed 25-Foot Walk is a quantitative measure of lower extremity function. It is the first component of the MSFC administered at each visit. The patient is directed to one end of a clearly marked 25-foot course and is instructed to walk 25 feet as quickly as possible, but safely. The task is immediately administered again by having the patient walk back the same distance. Patients may use assistive devices when doing this task. In clinical trials, it is recommended that the treating neurologist select the appropriate assistive device for each patient.

MATERIALS NEEDED
Stopwatch, clipboard, Timed 25-Foot Walk Record Form, marked 25-foot distance in an unobstructed hallway, assistive device (if needed)

TIME LIMIT PER TRIAL
3 minutes (180 seconds) per trial.

DISCONTINUE RULES
1. If the patient cannot complete Trial 2 of the Timed Walk after a 5-minute rest period.
2. If the patient cannot complete a trial in 3 minutes.

ADMINISTRATION
Administration of the Timed 25-Foot Walk is demonstrated on the training videotape.

Trial 1

Make sure that the stopwatch is set to 0:00. For the Timed 25-Foot Walk, the subject should be directed to one end of a clearly marked 25-foot course (clearly defined on the floor or on the wall) and instructed to stand just behind the starting line. Point out where the 25-foot course ends, then instruct the patient as follows: *'I'd like you to walk 25 feet as quickly as possible, but safely. Do not slow down until after you've passed the finish line. Ready? Go.'*

Begin timing when the lead foot is lifted and crosses the starting line. The examiner should walk along with the patient as he/she completes the task. Stop timing when the lead foot crosses the finish line. The examiner should then record the subject's walk time to within 0.1 second, rounding as needed. Round up to the next tenth if hundredth's place is ≤0.05, round down if hundredth's place is < 0.05 (e.g., 32.45" would round to 32.5" but 32.44" would round to 32.4"). Once the time is recorded, be sure to reset the stopwatch.

Trial 2

After completing the first timed walk, position the patient just behind the line where s/he is now standing, repeat the same instructions, and have the patient complete the walk again.

Assistive Devices

In clinical trials and other serial studies, the goal is to use the same assistive device at each study visit. The treating neurologist should select an assistive device at the beginning of the study for each patient who needs one, keeping in mind that the patient may deteriorate modestly over the course of a trial. In general, patients should use their customary assistive device(s), NOT the least assistance possible to complete the test. For patients with significant gait impairment, the treating neurologist should have the patient use a rolling walker even if this is not the patient's customary device. In general, non-wheeled walkers should *not* be used. If a patient does use an assistive device, this should be noted on the Record Form.

Completing the Record Form

Record any circumstances that you believe may have affected the patient's performance. These are factors that may have affected the trial but were not severe enough to necessitate repetition of the trial. Examples include, but are not limited to, the following:

- The patient had a cold or reports not feeling well.
- The patient tripped but did not fall.

If a situation arises that necessitates the repetition of a trial, indicate the reason a trial had to be repeated on the Record Form. Examples of reasons to repeat a trial include, but are not limited to, the following:

– The patient fell during the walk.
– Examiner forgot to start or stop stopwatch.
– Examiner forgot to reset stopwatch in between trials.
– The patient stopped to talk to someone while walking, or another person/thing somehow interfered with walk.

Record only the times for the two **successfully completed** trials of the Timed 25-Foot Walk. If the patient could not complete one or both of the trials of the Timed 25-Foot Walk, record this in the appropriate section of the Record Form. For example, if the patient's disease has progressed and/or physical limitations prohibit him or her from completing the trial, you should indicate 'Unable to complete trial due to physical limitations', and record any specifics that you can observe (i.e., patient in a wheelchair now and unable to walk, etc.). If the patient did not complete a trial for any other reason, specify this as well (e.g., patient fell and was too fatigued to complete another trial; patient refused to complete trial).

QUESTIONS ABOUT THE TIMED 25-FOOT WALK

Q. *Does it matter what kind of shoes the patient wears?*
A. As long as the style of the shoe is consistent for each patient from visit to visit, it does not matter what kind of shoes are worn. Encourage the patient to wear comfortable shoes and discourage patients from wearing, for example, high-heeled shoes one visit and running shoes the next.

Q. *Is the patient allowed to pause while walking the 25-foot distance?*
A. The patient should be encouraged to walk at a steady pace, one that he or she can sustain for 25 feet. However, pauses are allowed as long as the patient can complete the walk within the 3-minute time limit.

Q. *Is the patient allowed to run?*
A. No. The patient is to walk quickly but should not run.

Q. *Is the patient allowed to wear an AFO (ankle-foot orthosis) during the Timed 25-Foot Walk?*
A. If the patient typically wears an AFO and wears it every time the Timed

25-Foot Walk is performed, the patient may wear his/her AFO. Be sure to record this on the Record Form.

Q. *What should I do if the patient wants to use the wall as support while walking?*

A. The patient is only allowed to use customary assistive devices while walking (e.g., crutch, cane, wheeled walker, rollator) and therefore is not allowed to use a wall for continued support during the Timed 25-Foot Walk.

Q. *What should I do if the patient asks to lean on me for support while walking?*

A. This also is not allowed. Only customary assistive devices should be used if the patient needs extra support while walking.

Q. *How many times is the patient allowed to touch the wall or my arm momentarily for support during the walk?*

A. The patient is allowed to touch the wall or your arm a maximum of two times. If he or she touches the wall/your arm more than twice, repeat the trial, emphasizing to the patient that he or she is to walk using only the support of an assistive device. If the patient does not use an assistive device, notify the study coordinator that the patient may need to be reevaluated for use of an assistive device.

Q. *What's the difference between a cane and a crutch?*

A. A crutch extends under the axilla or supports the upper arm whereas the patient merely holds onto a cane.

Q. *What should I do if the patient drops his or her cane (or other assistive device) while walking?*

A. Restart the trial and record on the source document form.

Q. *Non-wheeled walkers are not allowed. What should I do if this is the assistive device the patient typically uses?*

A. Supply the patient with an accepted assistive device to use for the study visits. If it is a device unfamiliar to the patient, time should be allowed to practice with the device before the Timed 25-Foot Walk is administered.

Q. *It is standard practice at my site to use a guard belt during tasks such as the Timed 25-Foot Walk. Is that O.K. for this study?*

A. If this is standard practice for your site and all patients will consistently wear the guard belt for all trials of the Timed 25-Foot Walk for every visit, then this is acceptable. The device should neither assist nor encumber the patient.

Q. *Is it O.K. if the patient carries his/her purse or coat while he/she is walking?*

A. The patient should walk unencumbered. Patients should not be carrying any of their belongings during the Timed 25-Foot Walk. Furthermore, coats, purses, etc. should not be draped over wheeled walkers or rollators while the patient is completing the Timed 25-Foot Walk.

Q. *What should I do if the patient falls while s/he is walking?*

A. If the patient has not injured him/herself and is able to continue, start the trial over, reading the full instructions again. Emphasize that the patient should walk as quickly as possible, but *safely*. Record that the trial was repeated on the Record Form.

Q. *The patient keeps falling during the walk. How many attempted trials are permitted before I should discontinue and indicate that the patient was unable to complete the trial?*

A. Two. If the patient cannot successfully complete one trial of the Timed 25-Foot Walk in two consecutive attempts, discontinue the trial. Be sure to indicate this on the source document form.

Q. *What should I do if I forgot to reset the stopwatch between trials?*

A. If the stopwatch was not reset to 0:00, the trial will have to be repeated. On the Timed 25-Foot Walk Record Form, note that the trial was repeated and why.

INSTRUCTIONS FOR THE 9-HOLE PEG TEST (9-HPT)

DESCRIPTION

The 9-HPT is a quantitative measure of upper extremity (arm and hand) function. Its use with MS patients was first reported by Goodkin, Hertsgaard, & Seminary in 1988 (7), and it has seen increasing use in MS clinical trials and clinical practice during the last decade. The 9-HPT is the second component of the MSFC to be administered. Both the dominant and non-dominant hands are tested twice (two consecutive trials of the dominant hand, followed immediately by two consecutive trials of the non-dominant hand). It is important that the 9-HPT be administered on a solid table (not a rolling hospital bedside table) and that the 9-HPT apparatus be anchored (e.g., with Dycem).

MATERIALS NEEDED

9-HPT Apparatus, Dycem, stopwatch, clipboard, 9-HPT Record Form

TIME LIMIT PER TRIAL
5 minutes (300 seconds)

DISCONTINUE RULES
1. If the patient cannot complete one trial of the 9-HPT in 5 minutes.
2. If the patient cannot complete a trial with his or her dominant hand within 5 minutes, move on to the trials with the non-dominant hand.
3. If the patient cannot complete a trial with his or her non-dominant hand, move on to the PASAT.

ADMINISTRATION
Administration of the 9-HPT is demonstrated on the videotape

Dominant Hand—Trial 1
Make sure that the stopwatch is set to '0:00.' Introduce this section by saying, *'Now, we're going to be measuring your arm and hand function.'* If this is the first visit, ask, *'Are you right- or left-handed?'* Make a note of the dominant hand for subsequent instructions. Place the 9-HPT apparatus on the table directly in front of the patient. Arrange the apparatus so that the side with the pegs is in front of the hand being tested and the side with the empty pegboard is in front of the hand not being tested. Secure with Dycem.

Read the following instructions to the patient: *'On this test, I want you to pick up the pegs one at a time, using one hand only, and put them into the holes as quickly as you can in any order until all the holes are filled. Then, without pausing, remove the pegs one at a time and return them to the container as quickly as you can. We'll have you do this two (2) times with each hand. We'll start with your [DOMINANT] hand. You can hold the pegboard steady with your [NON-DOMINANT] hand. If a peg falls onto the table, please retrieve it and continue with the task. If a peg falls on the floor, keep working on the task and I will retrieve it for you. See how fast you can put all of the pegs in and take them out again. Are you ready? Begin.'*

Start timing as soon as the patient touches the first peg, and stop timing when the last peg hits the container. If a peg drops on the floor, the examiner may retrieve it and put it back in the peg box. However, if a peg drops onto the table, allow the patient to retrieve it.

Record the patient's time under 'Dominant hand—Trial 1.' If the subject stops after having put all the pegs into the holes, prompt the subject to remove them as well by saying, *'And now remove them all.'* If the subject begins to remove more than one peg at a time, correct him/her by saying, *'Pick up one peg at a time.'*

Dominant Hand—Trial 2

After the first trial with the dominant hand, say, 'Good. Now, I'd like you to do the same thing again, once again using your [DOMINANT] hand. See how fast you can put all of the pegs in and take them out again. Ready? Begin.' Again, start timing as soon as the patient touches the first peg, and stop timing when the last peg hits the container. Record the patient's time under 'Dominant hand—Trial 2.'

Non-Dominant Hand—Trials 1 and 2

After the second trial with the dominant hand, rotate the apparatus 180 degrees such that the side with the pegs is now in front of the non-dominant hand and the empty pegboard is in front of the dominant hand. Then say, *'O.K. Now I'd like you to switch and use your [NON-DOMINANT] hand. This time, you can use your [DOMINANT] hand to stabilize the pegboard. Ready? Begin.'* Administer, time, and record the two non-dominant hand trials following the procedures described above for dominant hand trials.

Completing the Record Form

Record any circumstances that you believe may have affected the patient's performance. These are factors that may have affected the trial, but were not severe enough to necessitate repetition of the trial. Examples include (but are not limited to) the following:

- The patient dropped a peg
- The patient has a cold
- The patient forgot eyeglasses and had difficulty seeing pegs
- The patient talked during the task

If a trial is repeated, indicate this and specify the reason it had to be repeated. Examples of reasons to repeat a trial include the following:

- The patient knocked entire apparatus on the floor
- The examiner forgot to start or stop stopwatch
- The examiner forgot to reset the stopwatch in between trials

Record only the times for the two **successfully completed** trials for each hand on the 9-HPT. If the patient could not complete one or both of the trials for either hand of the 9-HPT, record this in the appropriate section of the Record Forum. If the patient's disease has progressed and/or physical limitations prohibit him or her from completing the trial, the examiner should mark 'Unable to complete trial due to physical limitations,' and then record any specifics that can be observed (e.g., patient unable to use right hand, patient could not complete within time limit, etc.). If the patient did not complete a trial for any other reason, describe the specific circumstances (e.g., patient refused).

QUESTIONS ABOUT THE 9-HOLE PEG TEST

Q. *Is the patient allowed to take a break between the Timed Walk and the 9-HPT?*

A. Yes, but the patient is only allowed to rest a maximum of 5 minutes after the Timed Walk before starting the 9-HPT.

Q. *How should I determine the dominant hand if the patient indicates that he or she uses both hands?*

A. The dominant hand is the hand with which the patient writes (or did write) the majority of the time.

Q. *What should I do if the patient talks during the 9-HPT?*

A. Discourage the patient from talking as he or she completes the 9-HPT. You may quickly prompt the patient to remain quiet while the trial is in progress. Then, in between trials, emphasize to the patient that his or her concentration should be centered on the 9-HPT and that s/he should wait until the test is over to talk with you.

Q. *What should I do if a patient attempts to use both hands to complete a trial of the 9-HPT?*

A. Prompt the patient to use only one hand (dominant or non-dominant accordingly). If the patient continues to use both hands, start the trial over, emphasizing to the patient that s/he is to use only the one hand being tested.

Q. *What should I do if the patient takes out two pegs at a time?*

A. Prompt the patient with, 'Pick up one peg at a time.' If the patient responds to the prompt, and subsequently takes only one peg at a time, continue with the trial. If the patient continues to take out two pegs at a time, start the trial over, emphasizing to the patient that he/she must only pick up the pegs one at a time. Record the reason for the repeated trial on the Record Form.

Q. *What should I do if the patient takes more than two pegs at a time or even a whole handful of pegs at once?*

A. If the patient takes more than two pegs at a time, start the trial over, emphasizing that he/she must pick up only one peg at a time. Record the reason for the repeated trial on the Record Form.

Q. *What should I do if the patient knocks a peg out of a hole once it has already been placed?*

A. If a peg comes out of a hole and falls onto the table, let the patient retrieve it. If the peg comes out of a hole and falls onto the floor, you should retrieve it and place it in the container.

Q. *What should I do if the patient knocks the whole 9-HPT apparatus on the floor?*

A. Stop the trial. Reassemble the apparatus, repeat the instructions, and start the trial over. Encourage the patient to hold the pegboard steady with the hand he/she is not using, if possible. Note the incident in the appropriate section of the Record Form.

Q. *What should I do if the patient cannot complete the 9-HPT with one hand?*

A. If this happens on the enrollment visit (Day 1), the patient will not be able to enroll in the study. If this occurs once the patient is already enrolled in the study, indicate this in the appropriate section of the Record Form. Administer the 9-HPT at every visit, even if the patient was unable to complete it the visit before; the patient may be able to complete the test at subsequent visits.

Q. *Is the patient allowed to rest in between trials of the 9-HPT?*

A. No. The patient should progress directly from trial to trial, pausing only while you read the instructions for each subsequent trial.

Q. *What should I do if I forgot to reset the stopwatch in between trials?*

A. If the stopwatch was not reset to 0:00 at the beginning of the trial, that trial will have to be repeated. Note on the Record Form which trial(s) was repeated and why.

Q. *What should I do if I forgot to turn the 9-HPT apparatus when switching to the non-dominant hand?*

A. Start the trial over and note the reason for the repeated trial on the Record Form.

Q. *What should I do if I realize the 9-HPT kit is missing pegs?*

A. A supply of extra pegs can be ordered through the vendor. It is the examining technician's responsibility to make sure that all equipment is complete and in good working order prior to a study visit.

INSTRUCTIONS FOR THE PACED AUDITORY SERIAL ADDITION TEST (PASAT)

DESCRIPTION

The PASAT is a measure of cognitive function that specifically assesses auditory information processing speed and flexibility, as well as calculation ability. It was initially developed by Gronwall in 1977 to monitor the recovery of patients who had sustained concussions. It has been widely used in studies of head-injured patients over the last 20 years. Stimulus presentation rates were adapted for use with MS patients by Rao and colleagues in 1989, and the measure has been widely used in MS studies during the last decade. The PASAT is the last measure administered at each visit. It is presented on audiotape to control the rate of stimulus presentation. Single digits are presented every 3" (or every 2" for the optional 2" PASAT) and the patient must add each new digit to the one immediately prior to it. The test result is the number of correct sums given (out of 60 possible). To minimize familiarity with stimulus items in clinical trials and other serial studies, two alternate forms have been developed; the order of these should be counterbalanced across testing sessions.

MATERIALS NEEDED

Audiocassette tape player, audiocassette tape with PASAT stimuli, clipboard, PASAT Record Forms

DISCONTINUE RULES

1. If the patient cannot get at least two answers correct (consecutive or not) on any one of the three 3" practice sequences.
2. If the patient cannot get at least one answer correct on PASAT-3" test, do not administer the 2" test. This patient is considered unable to perform the test.

ADMINISTRATION

Administration of the PASAT is demonstrated on training videotape.

Verify that you have the correct Record Form and audiocassette (Form A or B) *before* you start reading the instructions for the 3" Practice Trial to the patient.

PASAT-3" Practice Trials

For Part 1 (stimuli every 3") say, *'On this tape you are going to hear a series of single digit numbers that will be presented at the rate of one every 3 seconds.*

Listen for the first two numbers, add them up, and tell me your answer.
When you hear the next number, add it to the one you heard on the tape
right before it. Continue to add the next number to each preceding one.
Remember, you are not being asked to give me a running total, but rather the
sum of the last two numbers that were spoken on the tape.'

Then give the following example: *'For example, if the first two numbers*
were '5' and '7,' you would say '12.' If the next number were '3,' you would
say '10.' Then if the next number were '2,' you would say '5.' ' If the patient is
having difficulty understanding these instructions, write 5, 7, 3, and 2 on a
sheet of paper and repeat the instructions, demonstrating how the task is done.

Then say, *'This is a challenging task. If you lose your place, just jump right*
back in—listen for two numbers in a row and add them up and keep going.
There are some practice items at the beginning of the tape. Let's try those first.'
Play the sample items, stopping the tape after the last practice item. Repeat the
practice items, if necessary, until the subject understands the instructions (up to
three times). You should always administer *at least one* practice trial before
administering the actual test. If the patient begins to give you a running total,
stop the practice immediately and explain the task again, emphasizing that
he/she is not to give you a running total. Then start the practice items again from
the beginning. If the patient begins adding each number to the number two
previous to it, again stop the practice immediately, explain the correct way to do
the task, and start the practice items from the beginning. If the patient merely
makes a math error, do not stop the tape; continue with the practice items. After
two consecutive 'no responses,' prompt him/her to resume by saying, *'Jump back*
in with the next two numbers you hear.'

Administer the practice sequence a *maximum of three times*. Record answers
in the space provided on the back of the PASAT Record Form.

PASAT-3"

Once it is clear that the patient possesses sufficient understanding of the task,
begin Part 1. Before starting Part 1, remind him/her: *'Remember, if you get lost,*
just jump back in because I can't stop the test once it has begun.' Discourage
talking and oral calculations during the test; only the patient's answers should
be spoken out loud. The patient may need prompting to continue the test if
she/he gets lost. After five consecutive 'no responses,' redirect the patient
quickly by saying, *'Jump back in,'* but do not stop the tape.

Note: Some cognitive neuropsychologists also recommend completing
the PASAT 2" to provide additional information about cognitive function.
This can be added as an option after the PASAT 3". Instructions for the

PASAT 2" follow, although only the PASAT 3" is currently recommended for inclusion in the MSFC.

PASAT-2" Practice Trials

Before Part 2 (stimuli every 2") say, *'There is a second part to this test, identical to the first, except that the numbers will come a little faster, one every 2 seconds. Let's try some practice items.'* Emphasize that the patient's task is the same, but that it is important to try to get his/her answer out as quickly as possible so as to hear the next number spoken on the tape. Every visit, *at least one* 2" practice trial must be administered before administering the 2" test. Allow *up to three* practice trials.

PASAT-2"

After the practice items, proceed directly with the 2" administration. If the patient completed the 3" PASAT, the 2" version is to be administered regardless of the patient's performance on the 2" practice items.

Completing the PASAT Record Form

Circle all correct answers. Write in any incorrect responses in the space provided. Write 'NR' (for 'no response') when no response was given. If the patient corrects him/herself after giving a response, count the amended answer as the response. The *amended* response is the one that will be used in determining total correct, regardless of whether it was the correct or incorrect response. *Slash through the old response and write in 'SC' with a circle around it to indicate that the patient self-corrected.*

Each section of the PASAT has a maximum of 60 correct answers (i.e. 61 digits are presented for each part). Count the total number correct (number of circled answers) for PASAT-3" and record on both the PASAT Record Form and the Summary Score Sheet. Repeat the same scoring procedure for PASAT-2". (Additional scores can also be computed to examine patterns of responses on the PASAT, but these are beyond the scope of this manual.)

Finally, record any circumstances that you believe may have affected the patient's performance. These are factors that may have affected the trial, but were not severe enough to necessitate repetition of the trial. Examples include, but are not limited to, the following:

- Subtle noises outside of the testing room
- Patient reports frustration or mild distress
- Patient talked during test (other than to give answers)

If a trial must be repeated, indicate this and specify the reason why it had to be repeated. Examples of reasons to repeat a trial include, but are not limited to the following:

- Test interrupted (e.g. someone walked into the room or other major disturbance)
- Examiner error, such as starting the tape in the wrong place or using the wrong form.

Record only totals for the **successfully completed** PASAT-3" and PASAT-2".

If the patient is unable to perform the PASAT (i.e., cannot get at least two correct on any 3" practice and at least one correct on the test portion), the examiner should indicate 'Unable to complete due to cognitive limitations' and record any specific observations. If the patient did not complete a trial for any other reason, record the reasons for this as well (e.g., patient refused to complete test, examiner forgot to administer PASAT-2", etc.).

QUESTIONS ABOUT THE PACED AUDITORY SERIAL ADDITION TEST

Q. *Can I operate the tape player on batteries when administering the PASAT?*

A. No. You should always run the tape player on electric power to ensure that the rate of stimulus presentation is standardized.

Q. *What should I do if the patient does not respond at all on the PASAT practice?*

A. If the patient has not made a response to any of the first five stimulus items, stop the practice trial and explain the task again. Remind the patient to state his/her answers aloud. Do not count the five 'no responses' as one of the three practice trials. (This situation is likely to occur only on the patient's first visit, when the patient is not familiar with the task.)

Q. *If the patient has performed well on the PASAT in past visits, do I still have to administer the PASAT practice sequence?*

A. Yes. At least one practice trial for both the 3" and 2" PASAT must be administered at every study visit. Failure to administer the practice trial will invalidate the data.

Q. *What should I do if the patient refuses to do the PASAT practice sequence?*

A. The PASAT practice is an important part of the PASAT and of the overall MSFC. The practice sequence is *not* optional and should not be presented as such. Explain to the patient that he or she must be given at least one 3″ and 2″ practice every study visit to maintain consistency. Emphasize the benefits that the practice trial will have on preparing him/her for the task.

Q. *Am I allowed to provide the patient with helpful strategies for the PASAT?*

A. No. You are allowed to give the patient only the standard instructions. Further explanations are allowed if the patient is having difficulty understanding the test, but these should be general instructions, not specific strategies to improve the patient's score.

Q. *Is the patient allowed to perform the calculations out loud, for example, to say '3 1 9 is 12,' etc.?*

A. All calculations are to be done silently. Indicate to the patient that oral calculations could interfere with his or her performance. Discourage the patient from talking, except to provide his or her answer. Watch for this behavior during practice trials and correct it before proceeding to the actual test.

Q. *Is the patient allowed to 'write' on the table with his or her finger during the PASAT?*

A. No. Observe the patient during the practice trials for this behavior. Instruct the patient that all calculations are to be done in his or her head and that 'writing down' the numbers is not permitted.

Q. *Is the patient allowed to count on his or her fingers?*

A. No. Again, if this behavior is exhibited by the patient during the practice, explain that is not allowed and that all calculations must be done in the patient's head.

Q. *I had already started the PASAT test and the patient asked to start over. Is this OK?*

A. No. As the instructions indicate, once the PASAT test has begun, you cannot stop it even if the patient requests to do so. The only reasons that you would stop the PASAT test would be because of a major external disturbance, equipment failure/malfunction, or something of this nature.

Q. *What should I do if the patient refuses to do the PASAT?*

A. The PASAT is a primary component of the MS Functional Composite. If a patient is unwilling to complete the PASAT, s/he may need to reconsider whether s/he wants to participate in the study.

Q. *Is the patient allowed to rest in between the PASAT 3″ and the PASAT 2″?*

A. No. You should proceed directly from the end of the PASAT 3″ test into the two second sequence (i.e., 2″ instructions, 2″ practice, then 2″ test).

Appendix 5

THE GUY'S NEUROLOGICAL DISABILITY SCALE (GNDS)

INSTRUCTIONS

The scale is designed to assess disability in patients with multiple sclerosis. It has 12 separate categories each with an interview and scoring section. The total GNDS score is the sum of the 12 separate scores. The questions are directed to assess the disability in the previous one month.

1. COGNITIVE DISABILITY:

A. Interview:

Do you have any problems with your memory or your ability to concentrate and work things out?

□ yes   □ no

Do your family or friends think that you have such a problem?

□ yes   □ no

If the answer to either question is 'yes':
Do you need help from other people for planning your normal daily affairs, handling money or making decisions?

□ yes   □ no

If 'yes': (To the examiner)
Is the patient orientated in time, place and person?

□ yes, fully
□ yes, partially*
□ no, totally disorientated*

*If the patient is not fully orientated, all their answers should be verified by the main carer(s) whose answers should take precedence.

Reproduced by permission from Sharrack B, Hughes RAC. The Guy's Neurological Disability Scale (GNSD). *Multiple Sclerosis* 1999; 5: 223–33.

B. Scoring:

0—No cognitive problems.

1—Cognitive problems not noticeable to family or friends.

2—Cognitive problems noticeable to family or friends but not requiring help from others.

3—Cognitive problems requiring help from others for normal daily affairs; patient is fully orientated in time, place and person.

4—Cognitive problems requiring help from others for normal daily affairs; patient is not fully orientated.

5—Patient is completely disorientated in time, place and person.

2. MOOD DISABILITY:

A. Interview:

Have you been feeling anxious, irritable, depressed, or had any mood swings during the last month?

☐ yes ☐ no

Are you taking any medications for such problem

☐ yes ☐ no

If the answer to the first question is 'yes':

Has the problem affected your ability to do *any* of your usual daily activities such as work, housework, or normal social activity with family and friends?

☐ yes ☐ no

If 'yes':

Has this problem been severe enough to prevent you from doing *all* your usual activities?

☐ yes ☐ no

Have you been admitted to hospital for treatment of your mood problem during the last month?

☐ yes ☐ no

B. Scoring

0—No mood problems.

1—Asymptomatic on current drug treatment.

2—Mood problems present but not affecting the patient's ability to perform any of their usual daily activities.

3—Mood problems affecting the patient's ability to perform some of their usual daily activities.

4—Mood problems preventing the patients from doing all their usual daily activities.

5—Mood problems requiring inpatient management.

X—Unknown (please score as the mean of the cognitive and fatigue disability scores rounded the nearest integer).

3. VISUAL DISABILITY:

A. Interview:

Do you have any problems with your vision that can't be corrected with ordinary glasses?

☐ yes ☐ no

If 'yes':

Can you read ordinary newspaper print (with ordinary glasses if worn, but not magnifying lenses)?

☐ yes ☐ no

If 'no':

Can you read large newspaper print?

☐ yes ☐ no

If 'no':

Can you count your fingers if you hold your hand out in front of you?

☐ yes ☐ no

If 'no':

Can you see your hand if you move it in front of you?

☐ yes ☐ no

B. Scoring:

0—No visual problems.

1—Visual problems (blurred vision, diplopia, scotomas) but patient is still able to read ordinary newspaper print.

2—Unable to read ordinary newspaper print.

3—Unable to read large newspaper print.

4—Unable to count fingers if they hold their hand out in front of them.

5—Unable to see hand movement if they move their hand in front of them.

4. SPEECH AND COMMUNICATION DISABILITY:

A. Interview:
Do you have any problems with your speech?
> ☐ yes ☐ no

If 'yes':
Do you have to repeat yourself when speaking to your family or close friends?
> ☐ yes ☐ no

If 'yes':
Do you need to use sign language, or the help of your carer to make people understand you?
> ☐ yes ☐ no

If 'yes': (to the examiner)
Is the patient able to communicate effectively using these methods?
> ☐ yes ☐ no

B. Scoring:
0—No speech problems.
1—Speech problems which does not require the patient to repeat themselves when speaking to strangers.
2—Speech problems which require the patient to repeat themselves when speaking to strangers.
3—Speech problems which require the patient to repeat themselves when speaking to their family and close friends.
4—Speech problems making speech difficult to understand; patient is able to communicate effectively by using sign language or the help of their carers.
5—Speech problems making speech difficult to understand, patient is unable to communicate effectively by using sign language or the help of their carers.

5. SWALLOWING DISABILITY:

A. Interview:

Do you have to take care when swallowing solids or fluids?

    ☐ yes   ☐   no

If 'yes':

Do you have to take care when swallowing with most meals?

    ☐ yes   ☐   no

If 'yes':

Do you need a special diet such as soft or liquidated food to help with your swallowing?

    ☐ yes   ☐   no

If 'yes':

Do you choke with most meals?

    ☐ yes   ☐   no

If 'yes':

Do you have a feeding tube (nasogastric or gastronomy tube)?

    ☐ yes   ☐   no

B. Scoring:

0—No swallowing problems.

1—Needs to be careful when swallowing solids or liquids but not with most meals.

2—Needs to be careful when swallowing solids or liquids with most meals; patient is able to eat food of normal consistency.

3—Needs specially prepared food of modified consistency.

4—Tendency to choke with most meals.

5—Dysphagia requiring nasogastric or gastrostomy tube.

6. UPPER LIMB DISABILITY:

A. Interview:

Do you have any problems with your hands or arms?

☐ yes ☐ no

If 'yes':

Do you have any difficulty in doing any of your zips *or* buttons?

☐ yes ☐ no

If 'yes':

Are you able to do *all* of your zips *and* buttons without help?

☐ yes ☐ no

Do you have any difficulty in tying a bow in laces or strings?

☐ yes ☐ no

If 'yes':

Are you able to tie a bow in laces or strings without help?

☐ yes ☐ no

Do you have any difficulty washing *and* brushing your hair?

☐ yes ☐ no

If 'yes':

Are you able to wash *and* brush your hair without help?

☐ yes ☐ no

Do you have any difficulty feeding yourself?

☐ yes ☐ no

If 'yes':

Are you able to feed yourself without help?

☐ yes ☐ no

If unable to do any of the functions listed:

Can you use your hands or arms for any other function?

☐ yes ☐ no

B. Scoring

0—No upper limb problem.

1—Problems in one or both arms, not affecting the ability to do any of the functions listed.

2—Problems in one or both arms, affecting some but not preventing any of the functions listed.

3—Problems in one or both arms, affecting all or preventing one or two of the functions listed.

4—Problems in one or both arms preventing three or all of the functions listed.

5—Unable to use either arm for any purposeful movements.

7. LOWER LIMB DISABILITY:

A. Interview:

Do you have any problems with your walking?

     □ yes   □   no

If 'yes':

Do you use a walking aid?

     □ yes   □   no

If 'yes':

A. How do you *usually* get around outdoors?

        □   without aid

or □   with one stick or crutch *or* holding on to someone's arm

or □   with two sticks or crutches *or* one stick or crutch and holding on to someone's arm

or □   with a wheelchair

B. How do you *usually* get around indoors?

        □   without aid

or □   with one stick or crutch *or* holding on to someone's arm

or □   with two sticks or crutches *or* one stick or crutch and holding on to someone's arm

or □   with a wheelchair

If you use a wheelchair:

Can you stand and walk a few steps with help?

     □ yes   □   no

B. Scoring

0—Walking is not affected.

1—Walking is affected but patient is able to walk independently.

2—Usually uses unilateral support (single stick or crutch, one arm) to walk outdoors, but walks independently indoors.

3—Usually uses bilateral support (two sticks or crutches, frame, or two arms) to walk outdoors, *or* unilateral support (single stick or crutch, or one arm) to walk indoors.

4—Usually uses wheelchair to travel outdoors, *or* bilateral support (two sticks or crutches, frame, or two arms) to walk indoors.

5—Usually uses a wheelchair indoors.

8. BLADDER DISABILITY

A. Interview:

Do you have any problems with your bladder?

☐ yes ☐ no

Are you taking any medications for such problems?

☐ yes ☐ no

If the answer to the first question is 'yes':

Do you have to rush to the toilet, go frequently, or have difficulty in starting to pass urine?

☐ yes ☐ no

Have you been incontinent in the last month?

☐ yes ☐ no

If 'yes':

Have you been incontinent in the last week?

☐ yes ☐ no

If 'yes':

Have you been incontinent every day?

☐ yes ☐ no

Do you use a catheter to empty your bladder?

☐ yes ☐ no

Do you need a permanent catheter in the bladder, or (*for men only*) do you use a sheath to collect your urine?

☐ yes ☐ no

231

B. Scoring:

0—Normal bladder problems.

1—Asymptomatic on current drug treatment.

2—Urinary frequency, urgency, or hesitancy with no incontinence.

3—Occasional urinary incontinence (once or more during the last month but not every week)

or intermittent catheterisation without incontinence.

4—Frequent urinary incontinence (once a week or more during the last month but not daily)

or occasional urinary incontinence despite regular intermittent catheterisation.

5—Daily urinary incontinence or permanent catheter (urethral/suprapubic) or penile sheath.

9. BOWEL DISABILITY:

A. Interview:

Do you have any problems with your bowel movements?

  ☐ yes   ☐   no

Are you on any medicines for such problems?

  ☐ yes   ☐   no

If the answer to the first question is 'yes':
Do you suffer with constipation?

  ☐ yes   ☐   no

If 'yes':
Do you need to take any laxatives or use suppositories for this?

  ☐ yes   ☐   no

Do you usually use enemas?

  ☐ yes   ☐   no

Do you usually evacuate your stools manually?

  ☐ yes   ☐   no

Do you have to rush to the toilet to open your bowels?

  ☐ yes   ☐   no

Have you had bowel accidents (been incontinent of faeces) in the last week?

  ☐ yes   ☐   no

If 'yes':

Have you had bowel accidents every week?

☐ yes ☐ no

B. Scoring:

0—No bowel problems.

1—Asymptomatic on current drug treatment or constipation not requiring any treatment.

2—Constipation requiring laxatives or suppositories *or* faecal urgency.

3—Constipation requiring the use of enemas.

4—Constipation requiring manual evacuation of stools *or* occasional faecal incontinence (once or more during the last month but not every week).

5—Weekly faecal incontinence.

10. SEXUAL DISABILITIES:

A. Interview:

The next set of questions relates to sexual function. Do you mind if I ask you about this?

☐ yes

☐ no

☐ not applicable (Celibate)

If the patient agrees:

Do you have any problems in relation to your sexual function?

☐ yes ☐ no

If 'yes':

Do you suffer with lack of sexual interest?

☐ yes ☐ no

Do you have any problems satisfying yourself or your sexual partner?

☐ yes ☐ no

Is your sexual function affected by any physical problem such as altered genital sensation, pain, or spasms?

☐ yes ☐ no

Do you have any problems with:

(for men): erection/ejaculation?

(for women): vaginal lubrication/orgasm?

☐ yes ☐ no

If physical or sexual problems are present:
Do any of these difficulties totally prevent your sexual activities?
□ yes   □ no

B. Scoring:

0—Normal sexual functions *or* persons who are voluntarily celibate.
1—Reduced sexual interest.
2—Problems satisfying oneself or sexual partner.
3—Physical problems interfering but not preventing sexual function.
4—Autonomic problems interfering but not preventing sexual function.
5—Physical or autonomic problems totally preventing sexual function.
X—Unknown (please score as the mean of the lower limb, bladder, and bowel disability scores rounded to the nearest integer).

11. FATIGUE:

A. Interview:

Have you been feeling tired or getting tired easily during the last month?
□ yes   □ no

If 'yes':
Have you been feeling tired most days?
□ yes   □ no

Has this tiredness affected your ability to do *any* of your usual activities such as work, housework, or normal social activity with family and friends?
□ yes   □ no

If 'yes':
Has this tiredness been severe enough to prevent you from doing *all* of your usual activities?
□ yes   □ no

If 'yes':
Has the tiredness been severe enough to prevent you from doing *all* physical activities?
□ yes   □ no

B. Scoring:

0—Absent.
1—Occasional fatigue (present some days).
2—Frequent fatigue (present most days).

3—Fatigue affecting the patient's ability to perform some of their usual daily activities.

4—Fatigue preventing the patient from doing all their usual daily activities.

5—Fatigue preventing the patient from doing all their physical activities.

X—Unknown (please score as the mean of the cognitive and mood disability scores rounded to the nearest integer).

12. OTHER DISABILITIES:

A. Interview:

Do you have other problems due to MS such as pain, spasms, or dizziness which have not been mentioned so far?

☐ yes ☐ no

Are you taking any medicines for such problems?

☐ yes ☐ no

If the answer to either question is 'yes':

Please name your worst problem: ....

Has this problem affected your ability to do *any* of your usual daily activities?

☐ yes ☐ no

Has this problem been severe enough to prevent you from doing *all* your usual daily activities?

☐ yes ☐ no

Have you been admitted to hospital for treatment of this problem?

☐ yes ☐ no

B. Scoring:

0—Absent.

1—Asymptomatic on current drug treatment.

2—Problems, present, but are not affecting the patient's ability to perform any of their usual daily activities.

3—Problems affecting the patient's ability to perform some of their usual daily activities.

4—Problems preventing the patient from doing all their usual daily activities.

5—Problems requiring hospital admission for assessment or treatment.

Appendix 6

THE MOS 36-ITEM SHORT-FORM HEALTH SURVEY (SF-36)

I. CONCEPTUAL FRAMEWORK AND ITEM SELECTION

Appendix. SF-36 Questions[a]

1. In general, would you say your health is:

2. *Compared to one year ago*, how would you rate your health in general *now*?

3. The following items are about activities you might do during a typical day. Does *your health now limit you* in these activities? If so, how much?
   a. *Vigorous activities*, such as running, lifting heavy objects, participating in strenuous sports
   b. *Moderate activities*, such as moving a table, pushing a vacuum cleaner, bowling, or playing golf
   c. Lifting or carrying groceries
   d. Climbing *several* flights of stairs
   e. Climbing *one* flight of stairs
   f. Bending, kneeling, or stooping
   g. Walking *more than a mile*
   h. Walking *several blocks*
   i. Walking *one block*
   j. Bathing or dressing yourself

4. During the *past 4 weeks*, have you had any of the following problems with your work or other regular daily activities *as a result of your physical health*?
   a. Cut down the *amount of time* you spent on work or other activities.
   b. *Accomplished less* than you would like
   c. Were limited in the *kind* of work or other activities
   d. Had *difficulty* performing the work or other activities (for example, it took extra effort)

Reproduced by permission from Ware JE, Jr, Donald Sherbourne C. The MOS 36-Item Short Form Health Survey (SF36). *Med Care* 1992; 30: 473–83.

5. During the *past 4 weeks*, have you had any of the following problems with your work or other regular daily activities *as a result of any emotional problems* (such as feeling depressed or anxious)?
   a. Cut down the *amount of time* you spent on work or other activities
   b. *Accomplished less* than you would like
   c. Didn't do work or other activities as *carefully* as usual

6. During the *past 4 weeks*, to what extent has your physical health or emotional problems interfered with your normal social activities with family, friends, neighbors, or groups?

7. How much *bodily* pain have you had during the *past 4 weeks*?

8. During the *past 4 weeks*, how much did *pain* interfere with your normal work (including both work outside the home and housework)?

9. These questions are about how you feel and how things have been with you *during the past 4 weeks*. For each question, please give the one answer that comes closest to the way you have been feeling. How much of the time during the *past 4 weeks*
   a. Did you feel full of pep?
   b. Have you been a very nervous person?
   c. Have you felt so down in the dumps that nothing could cheer you up?
   d. Have you felt calm and peaceful?
   e. Did you have a lot or energy?
   f. Have you felt downhearted and blue?
   g. Did you feel worn out?
   h. Have you been a happy person?
   i. Did you feel tired?

10. During the *past 4 weeks*, how much of the time has your *physical health or emotional problems* interfered with your social activities (like visiting with friends, relatives, etc.)?

11. How TRUE or FALSE is *each* of the following statements for you?
    a. I seem to get sick a little easier than other people
    b. I am as healthy as anybody I know
    c. I expect my health to get worse
    d. My health is excellent

SF-36 Response Choices[a]

1. Excellent, Very Good, Good, Fair, Poor

2. Much better now than one year ago, Somewhat better now than one year ago, About the same as one year ago, Somewhat worse now than one year ago, Much worse than one year ago

3. Yes, Limited a lot; Yes, Limited a little; No, Not limited at all

4a–d. Yes, No

5a–c. Yes, No

6. Not at all, Slightly, Moderately, Quite a bit, Extremely

7. None, Very mild, Mild, Moderate, Severe, Very severe

8. Not at all, A little bit, Moderately, Quite a bit, Extremely

9. All of the time, Most of the time, A good bit of the time, Some of the time, A little of the time, None of the time

10. All of the time, Most of the time, Some of the time, A little of the time, None of the time

11. Definitely true, Mostly true, Don't know, Mostly false, Definitely false

Table 1 Information About SF-36 Health Status Scales and the Interpretation of Low and High Scores

Concepts	No. of Items	No. of Levels	Meaning of Scores	
			Low	High
Physical functioning	10	21	Limited a lot in performing all physical activities including bathing or dressing	Performs all types of physical activities including the most vigorous without limitations due to health
Role limitations due to physical problems	4	5	Problems with work or other daily activities as a result of physical health	No problems with work or other daily activities as a result of physical health, past 4 weeks
Social functioning	2	9	Extreme and frequent interference with normal social activities due to physical and emotional problems	Performs normal social activities without interference due to physical or emotional problems, past 4 weeks
Bodily pain	2	11	Very severe and extremely limiting pain	No pain or limitations due to pain, past 4 weeks
General mental health	5	26	Feelings of nervousness and depression all of the time	Feels peaceful, happy, and calm all of the time, past 4 weeks
Role limitations due to emotional problems	3	4	Problems with work or other daily activities as a result of emotional problems	No problems with work or other daily activities as a result of emotional problems, past 4 weeks
Vitality	4	21	Feels tired and worn out all of the time	Feels full of pep and energy all of the time, past 4 weeks
General health perceptions	5	21	Believes personal health is poor and likely to get worse	Believes personal health is excellent

Appendix 7

FARMER QUALITY OF LIFE SCALE

QOL SCALE

A QOL scale, the Farmer QOL Index (subsequently referred to as the QOL scale), was developed by one of us (R.G.F.) at The Cleveland (Ohio) Clinic Foundation in 1988. It was originally used with a population of patients with IBD. The QOL scale as originally published consists of 47 questions that are grouped into four clusters: (1) functional and economic subscale (12 questions), (2) social and recreational subscale (15 questions), (3) affect and life in general subscale (11 questions), and (4) medical problems subscale (nine questions).

The QOL scale was administered as a structured interview in which each question was posed with the response rated on a five-point scale. One end of the scale represented the best response and the other end represented the worst response. The direction of the response was varied in a standardized format in the interview; responses were subsequently reordered so that 1 always represented the worst response and 5 represented the best response. The entire QOL scale was then summed to render an overall score, and each subscale was independently summed to render subscale scores for each patient.

The QOL scale was with the elimination of six items. One question was deleted from the social and recreational subscale because the elicited response could not be coded on a five-point scale. Five questions were omitted from the medical problems subscale because they were not applicable to MS. Therefore, the QOL scale used consisted of 41 questions (Tables 1 through 5). The instrument required 15 to 30 minutes per patient to complete.

Table 1 Farmer Quality of Life Index – Subscale
Functional and economic
Social and recreational
Affect and life in general
Medical problems

Reproduced by permission from Rudick RA *et al*. Quality of Life in Multiple Sclerosis. *Arch Neurol* 1992; 49: 1237–42. © 1992 American Medical Association.

Table 2 Functional and Economic Subscale Questions

- I have been able to fulfill my educational goals
- I am able to support myself and my family
- I I am receiving financial support from a source other than employment
- I am having difficulty getting insurance
- I feel that I am able to get through each day as well as others
- My earnings are as good as others in similar jobs or activities
- My disease has made it difficult for me to obtain a job
- My symptoms interfere with my job or activities
- In comparing myself to others, I feel I have less energy
- I am able to carry out my regular activities in a way satisfying to me
- I feel I have been able to move ahead in my job and family responsibilities
- My growth and physical development were affected by my illness

Table 3 Social and Recreational Subscale Questions

- I am able to enjoy activities with my family
- I have someone to talk to about the way I feel
- I feel isolated because of my disease
- I canceled an activity this past month because of symptoms
- I feel frightened by the future
- I participate in social activities with friends
- I can depend on my family or friends for support
- I am able to participate in a recreational or sport activity regularly
- I belong and participate regularly in a club, church, or professional organization
- I feel satisfied with my relationship with my spouse or significant other
- I feel satisfied about the way I participate in family activities
- My disease has made it difficult for me to have a family
- My condition has made it difficult for me to share intimate relationships
- I participate in a hobby or special interest in addition to other tasks

Table 4 Affect and Life in General Subscale Questions

- I have made plans for things to do next month
- Most of the time I sleep through the night
- I have made plans for things I'll be doing a year from now
- My life is going along pretty much as I had planned
- When compared with other persons of my age, I feel pleased with my accomplishments
- I feel frustrated with my health problems
- I look forward to each day
- I frequently worry about my health
- In comparison to other people, I feel I become more easily discouraged
- I find that I need mood elevating medications to help get me through the day Others see me as chronically ill

Table 5 Medical Problems Subscale Questions

- I would describe my general physical condition in comparison to others as . . . (1, poor; 5, good)
- My symptoms significantly affect the way I function each day (1, constantly; 5, never)
- I take medications (1, regularly; 5, occasionally)
- I take prednisone at least once a day (1, yes; 2, no)

Appendix 8

MULTIPLE SCLEROSIS QUALITY OF LIFE (MSQOL)-54 INSTRUMENT

Key to final item placement into scales:

Scale	Item numbers
Physical health	3–12*
Role limitations due to physical problems	13–16*
Role limitations due to emotional problems	17–19*
Pain	21*, 22*, 52
Emotional well-being	24–26*, 28*, 30*
Energy	23*, 27*, 29*, 31*, 32
Health perceptions	1*, 34–37*
Social function	20*, 33*, 51
Cognitive function	42–45
Health distress	38–41
Overall quality of life	53–54
Sexual function	46–49
Change in health	2*
Satisfaction with sexual function	50

*Indicates SF-36 (or RAND 36-Item Health Survey 1.0) item. This measure was developed based on research conducted for the Health Insurance Experiment and the Medical Outcomes Study, carried out at RAND and funded by a variety of federal and private agencies. There are minor differences in scoring the two measures;[19] permission for use may be obtained by writing the Medical Outcomes Trust (Boston, Massachusetts) for the SF-36, and RAND (Santa Monica, California) for the RAND 36-Item Health Survey.

Reproduced by permission from Vickrey BG *et al*. A health-related quality of life measure for multiple sclerosis. *Quality of Life Research* 1995; 4: 187–206. With kind permission of Kluwer Academic Publishers.

INSTRUCTIONS:

This survey asks about your health and daily activities. *Answer every question* by circling the appropriate number (1, 2, 3, . . .).

If you are unsure about how to answer a question, please give the best answer you can and write a comment or explanation in the margin.

Please feel free to ask someone to assist you if you need help reading or marking the form.

1. In general would you say your health is:

(circle one number)

Excellent 1

Very good 2

Good 3

Fair 4

Poor 5

2. *Compared to one year ago*, how would you rate your health in general *now*?

(circle one number)

Much better now than one year ago 1

Somewhat better now than one year ago . . 2

About the same 3

Somewhat worse now than one year ago . . 4

Much worse now than one year ago 5

3–12. The following questions are about activities you might do during a typical day. Does *your health* limit you in these activities? If so, how much?

(Circle 1, 2 or 3 on each line)

	Yes, limited a lot	Yes, limited a little	No, not limited at all
3. *Vigorous activities*, such as running, lifting heavy objects, participating in strenuous sports	1	2	3
4. *Moderate activities*, such as moving a table, pushing a vacuum cleaner, bowling, or playing golf	1	2	3
5. Lifting or carrying groceries	1	2	3
6. Climbing *several* flights of stairs	1	2	3
7. Climbing *one* flight of stairs	1	2	3
8. Bending, kneeling or stooping	1	2	3
9. Walking *more than a mile*	1	2	3
10. Walking *several blocks*	1	2	3
11. Walking *one block*	1	2	3
12. Bathing and dressing yourself	1	2	3

13–16. During the *past 4 weeks*, have you had any of the following problems with your work or other regular daily activities *as a result of your physical health*?

(Circle one number on each line)

	YES	NO
13. Cut down on the *amount of time* you could spend on work or other activities	1	2
14. *Accomplished less* than you would like	1	2
15. Were limited in the *kind* of work or other activities	1	2
16. Had *difficulty* performing the work or other activities	1	2

17–19. During the *past 4 weeks*, have you had any of the following problems with your work or other regular daily activities *as a result of any emotional problems* (such as feeling depressed or anxious).

(Circle one number on each line)

	YES	NO
17. Cut down on the *amount of time* you could spend on work or other activities	1	2
18. *Accomplished less* than you would like	1	2
19. Didn't do work or other activities as *carefully* as usual	1	2

20. During the *past 4 weeks*, to what extent has your physical health or emotional problems interfered with your normal social activities with family, friends, neighbors or groups?

(circle one number)

Not at all 1

Slightly 2

Moderately 3

Quite a bit 4

Extremely 5

Pain

21. How much *bodily* pain have you had during the *past 4 weeks*?

(circle one number)

None 1

Very mild 2

Mild 3

Moderate 4

Severe 5

Very severe 6

22. During the *past 4 weeks*, how much did *pain* interfere with your normal work (including both work outside the home and housework)?

(circle one number)

Not at all 1

A little bit 2

Moderately 3

Quite a bit 4

Extremely 5

23–32. These questions are about how you feel and how things have been with you *during the past 4 weeks*. For each question, please give the one answer that comes closest to the way you have been feeling.

How much of the time during the *past 4 weeks* . . .

(Circle one number on each line)

	All of the time	Most of the time	A good bit of the time	Some of the time	A little of the time	None of the time
23. Did you feel full of pep?	1	2	3	4	5	6
24. Have you been a very nervous person?	1	2	3	4	5	6
25. Have you felt so down in the dumps that nothing could cheer you up?	1	2	3	4	5	6
26. Have you felt calm and peaceful?	1	2	3	4	5	6
27. Did you have a lot of energy?	1	2	3	4	5	6
28. Have you felt downhearted and blue?	1	2	3	4	5	6
29. Did you feel worn out?	1	2	3	4	5	6
30. Have you been a happy person?	1	2	3	4	5	6
31. Did you feel tired?	1	2	3	4	5	6
32. Did you feel rested on waking in the morning?	1	2	3	4	5	6

33. During the *past 4 weeks*, how much of the time has your *physical health or emotional problems* interfered with your social activities (like visiting with friends, relatives, etc.)?

(circle one number)

Not at all 1

A little bit 2

Moderately 3

Quite a bit 4

Extremely 5

Health in General

34–37. How TRUE or FALSE is *each* of the following statements for you.
(Circle one number on each line)

	Definitely true	Mostly true	Not sure	Mostly false	Definitely false
34. I seem to get sick a little easier than other people	1	2	3	4	5
35. I am as healthy as anybody I know	1	2	3	4	5
36. I expect my health to get worse	1	2	3	4	5
37. My health is excellent	1	2	3	4	5

Health Distress

38–41. How much of the time during the *past 4 weeks* . . .
(Circle one number on each line)

	All of the time	Most of the time	A good bit of the time	Some of the time	A little of the time	None of the time
38. Were you discouraged by your health problems?	1	2	3	4	5	6
39. Were you frustrated about your health?	1	2	3	4	5	6
40. Was your health a worry in your life?	1	2	3	4	5	6
41. Did you feel weighed down by your health problems?	1	2	3	4	5	6

Cognitive function

42–45. How much of the time during the *past 4 weeks* . . .
(Circle one number on each line)

	All of the time	Most of the time	A good bit of the time	Some of the time	A little of the time	None of the time
42. Have you had difficulty concentrating and thinking?	1	2	3	4	5	6
43. Did you have trouble keeping your attention on an activity for long?	1	2	3	4	5	6
44. Have you had trouble with your memory?	1	2	3	4	5	6
45. Have others, such as family members or friends, noticed that you have trouble with your memory or problems with your concentration?	1	2	3	4	5	6

Sexual function

46–49. The next set of questions are about your sexual function and your satisfaction with your sexual function. Please answer as accurately as possible about your function *during the last 4 weeks only*.

How much of a problem was each of the following for you *during the past 4 weeks*?

(Circle one number on each line)

Men	Not a problem	A little of a problem	Somewhat of a problem	Very much a problem
46. Lack of sexual interest	1	2	3	4
47. Difficulty getting or keeping an erection	1	2	3	4
48. Difficulty having orgasm	1	2	3	4
49. Ability to satisfy sexual partner	1	2	3	4

(Circle one number on each line)

Women	Not a problem	A little of a problem	Somewhat of a problem	Very much a problem
46. Lack of sexual interest	1	2	3	4
47. Difficulty getting or keeping an erection	1	2	3	4
48. Difficulty having orgasm	1	2	3	4
49. Ability to satisfy sexual partner	1	2	3	4

50. Overall, how satisfied were you with your sexual function *during the past 4 weeks*?

(circle one number)

Very satisfied 1

Somewhat satisfied .2

Neither satisfied nor dissatisfied 3

Somewhat dissatisfied 4

Very dissatisfied 5

51. During the *past 4 weeks*, to what extent have problems with your bowel or bladder function interfered with your normal social activities with family, friends, neighbors or groups?

(circle one number)

Not at all 1

Slightly 2

Moderately 3

Quite a bit 4

Extremely 5

52. During the *past 4 weeks*, how much did *pain* interfere with your enjoyment of life?

(circle one number)

Not at all 1

Slightly 2

Moderately 3

Quite a bit 4

Extremely 5

QUALITY OF LIFE

53. Overall, how would you rate your own quality-of-life?

Circle one number on the scale below:

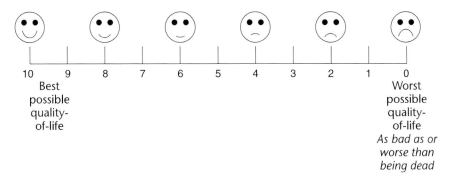

54. Which best describes how you feel about your life as a whole?

(circle one number)

Terrible 1

Unhappy 2

Mostly dissatisfied 3

Mixed—about equally satisfied and
dissatisfied 4

Mostly satisfied 5

Pleased 6

Delighted 7

Appendix 9

THE FAMS QUALITY OF LIFE INSTRUMENT

Discussion. The FAMS quality of life instrument is a 59-item multidimensional index of health-related quality of life (FAMS version 2) for use with people diagnosed with MS. Forty-four items are used for scoring purposes.

Appendix FAMS (Version 2). *Below is a list of statements that other people with your illness have said are important. By circling one number per line, please indicate how true each statement has been for you during the past 7 days.*

Mobility	not at all	a little bit	some- what	quite a bit	very much
1. Because of my physical condition, I have trouble meeting the needs of my family	0	1	2	3	4
2. I am able to work (include work in home)	0	1	2	3	4
3. I have trouble walking	0	1	2	3	4
4. I have to limit my social activity because of my condition	0	1	2	3	4
5. My legs are strong	0	1	2	3	4
6. I have trouble getting around in public places	0	1	2	3	4
7. I have to make plans around my condition	0	1	2	3	4

Symptoms	not at all	a little bit	some- what	quite a bit	very much
8. I have nausea	0	1	2	3	4
9. I have pain	0	1	2	3	4
10. I feel sick	0	1	2	3	4
11. I feel weak all over	0	1	2	3	4
12. I have pain in my joints	0	1	2	3	4
13. I am bothered by headaches	0	1	2	3	4
14. I am bothered by muscle pains	0	1	2	3	4

Emotional Well-Being	not at all	a little bit	some-what	quite a bit	very much
15. I feel sad	0	1	2	3	4
16. I am losing hope in the fight against my illness	0	1	2	3	4
17. I am able to enjoy life	0	1	2	3	4
18. I feel trapped by my condition	0	1	2	3	4
19. I am depressed about my condition	0	1	2	3	4
20. I feel useless	0	1	2	3	4
21. I feel overwhelmed by my condition	0	1	2	3	4

Please indicate how true each statement has been for you during the past 7 days.

General Contentment	not at all	a little bit	some-what	quite a bit	very much
22. My work (include work in home) is fulfilling	0	1	2	3	4
23. I have accepted my illness	0	1	2	3	4
24. I am enjoying the things I usually do for fun	0	1	2	3	4
25. I am content with the quality of my life right now	0	1	2	3	4
26. I am frustrated by my condition	0	1	2	3	4
27. I feel a sense of purpose in my life	0	1	2	3	4
28. I feel motivated to do things	0	1	2	3	4

Thinking and Fatigue	not at all	a little bit	some-what	quite a bit	very much
29. I have a lack of energy	0	1	2	3	4
30. I feel tired	0	1	2	3	4
31. I have trouble *starting* things because I am tired	0	1	2	3	4
32. I have trouble *finishing* things because I am tired	0	1	2	3	4
33. I need to rest during the day	0	1	2	3	4
34. I have trouble remembering things	0	1	2	3	4
35. I have trouble concentrating	0	1	2	3	4
36. My thinking is slow	0	1	2	3	4
37. I have trouble learning new tasks or directions	0	1	2	3	4

Family/Social Well-Being	not at all	a little bit	some- what	quite a bit	very much
38. I feel distant from my friends	0	1	2	3	4
39. I get emotional support from my family	0	1	2	3	4
40. I get support from my friends and neighbors	0	1	2	3	4
41. My family has accepted my illness	0	1	2	3	4
42. Family communication about my illness is poor	0	1	2	3	4
43. My family has trouble understanding when my condition gets worse	0	1	2	3	4
44. I feel 'left out' of things	0	1	2	3	4

Please indicate how true each statement has been for you during the past 7 days.

Additional Concerns	not at all	a little bit	some- what	quite a bit	very much
45. I am bothered by side effects of treatment	0	1	2	3	4
46. I am forced to spend time in bed	0	1	2	3	4
47. I feel close to my partner (or the person who is my main support)	0	1	2	3	4
48. Have you been sexually active during the past year? No__ Yes__ If yes: I am satisfied with my sex life	0	1	2	3	4
49. My doctor is available to answer my questions	0	1	2	3	4
50. I am proud of how I'm coping with my illness	0	1	2	3	4
51. I feel nervous	0	1	2	3	4
52. I worry that my condition will get worse	0	1	2	3	4
53. I am sleeping well	0	1	2	3	4
54. Heat worsens my symptoms	0	1	2	3	4
55. I lose control of my urine	0	1	2	3	4
56. I urinate more frequently than usual	0	1	2	3	4
57. I am bothered by the chills	0	1	2	3	4
58. I am bothered by fevers	0	1	2	3	4
59. I am bothered by muscle spasms	0	1	2	3	4